DATE DUE

SEP 2 5 1995	DEC 1 8 2002
MAY 2 0 1996	MAY 2 0 2003
JAN 4 1997	NOV 1 9 2003
MAY 1 9 1997	
NOV 2 1997	DEC 2 2 2003
MAY 1 4 1998	MAY 1 3 2004
NOV 2 5 1998	
APR 2 7 1999	NOV 2 2 2005
NOV 2 - 1999	DEC 1 5 2008
DEC 1 6 1999	MAY 1 7 2009
FEB 2 1 2000	JUN 2 6 2010
JAN 2 2001	NOV 2 5 2010
APR 2 7 2001	
MAY 1 7 2001	APR 0 9 2018
DEC 9 - 2001	
DEC 5 - 2002	

Library of Congress Cataloging-in-Publication Data

Anabolic steroids in sport and exercise / Charles E. Yesalis, editor.
   p. cm
   Includes bibliographical references and index.
   ISBN 0-87322-401-9
   1. Anabolic steroids--Health aspects. 2. Doping in sports.
 I. Yesalis, Charles.
 RC1230.A522   1993
 362.29'08'8796--dc20

92-20143
CIP

ISBN: 0-87322-401-9

Acquisitions Editor: Rick Frey, PhD; **Developmental Editor**: Christine Drews; **Assistant Editors**: Julie Swadener, Valerie Hall, Laura Bofinger, and Dawn Roselund; **Copyeditor**: Julie Anderson; **Proofreader**: Kari Nelson; **Indexer**: Schroeder Indexing Services; **Production Director**: Ernie Noa; **Typesetting and Text Layout**: Yvonne Winsor, Angela K. Snyder, and Kathy Fuoss; **Text Design**: Keith Blomberg; **Cover Design**: Jack Davis; **Interior Art**: Tom Janowski; **Printer**: Braun-Brumfield, Inc.; **Photo credits**: p. xiii, University Photo/Graphics, The Pennsylvania State University; p. 1, Reuters/Bettmann Newsphotos; p. 87, John Kilroy/Photo Concepts; p. 251, courtesy of James Wright, PhD.

Printed in the United States of America   10 9 8 7 6 5 4 3

Human Kinetics
P.O. Box 5076, Champaign, IL 61825-5076
1-800-747-4457

Canada: Human Kinetics, Box 24040, Windsor, ON N8Y 4Y9
1-800-465-7301 (in Canada only)

Europe: Human Kinetics, P.O. Box IW14
Leeds LS16 6TR, England
0532-781708

Australia: Human Kinetics, P.O. Box 80, Kingswood 5062
South Australia
618-374-0433

New Zealand: Human Kinetics, P.O. Box 105-231, Auckland 1
(09) 309-2259

Perspectives on Steroid Use

For a great many years I have believed that the weakness of old men depended on two causes—a natural series of organic changes and the gradually diminishing action of the spermatic glands.

E.C. Brown-Séquard
Lancet, 1889 **(2)**

The use of artificial means [to improve performance] has long been considered wholly incompatible with the spirit of sport and has therefore been condemned. Nevertheless, we all know that this rule is continually being broken, and that sportive competitions are often more a matter of doping than of training. It is highly regrettable that those who are in charge of supervising sport seem to lack the energy for the campaign against this evil, and that a lax, and fateful, attitude is spreading. Nor are the physicians without blame for this state of affairs, in part on account of their ignorance, and in part because they are prescribing strong drugs for the purpose of doping which are not available to athletes without prescriptions.

O. Riesser
"Über Doping und Dopingmittel" in
Leibesübungen und körperliche Erziehung, 1933
Found in John M. Hoberman, Mortal Engines, 1992

Lie #1: Anabolic steroids do not enhance athletic performance.
Lie #2: Steroids will kill you.
Lie #3: You can get the same results without steroids, you just have to work longer and harder.

Dan Duchaine
Underground Steroid Handbook II, 1989

My definition of cheating is doing something nobody else is doing.

Charlie Francis
Former coach of Ben Johnson
Sports Illustrated, *December 17, 1990*

The major side effect of anabolic steroids is hypocrisy.

Tony Fitton
Six-time British power lifting champion

The State of the Game

I woke up this morning after a night of killing pain.
I went to the practice field to deal with it again.
My coach, he tells me, "Fight hard and be a man!"
But with his chalk board theories we all wonder if he can?
So knock 'em down, block 'em hard and strive to win the fight.
I wonder why they're so concerned, is it economic plight?
The battle in the trenches, won and lost, and who does realize
But the gladiator in its midst whose soul in anguish cries.
What keeps him in the arena but those fine and great ideals,
But it's become just a business, what matter how he feels.
The battle fought, the game is won, and victor duly glorified.
But the sad fact, businessman, is the sporting soul has died.
In the end in retrospect what's glorified and gained
But the almighty dollar, not the spirit of the game.

Steve Courson
Pittsburgh Steelers 1977-83
Tampa Bay Buccaneers 1984-85

Editor's Note

Although the proper term for the types of drugs discussed in this book is *anabolic-androgenic steroids* (see chapter 1), the more common terms *anabolic steroid* and *steroid* are often used for convenience.

To Diane and Steve,
who taught me the meaning of courage.

To Dan, Mark, and Ed,
who showed me what real intensity is.

Contributors

Editor

Charles E. Yesalis, ScD, received his master of public health degree from the University of Michigan and completed his doctoral work at the Johns Hopkins School of Hygiene and Public Health in 1975. Dr. Yesalis was a member of the Department of Preventive Medicine and Environmental Health at the University of Iowa, College of Medicine, from 1976 to 1986. Currently, he is a professor of health policy and administration and exercise and sport science at The Pennsylvania State University.

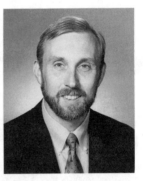

Dr. Yesalis directed the first national study of anabolic steroid use among adolescents and was the first to present evidence of psychological dependence on anabolic steroids. On three occasions he has been asked to testify before U.S. Congress on legislation related to the control of anabolic steroid and growth hormone abuse.

Contributors

Michael S. Bahrke received his MS in exercise physiology and his PhD in sport psychology from the University of Wisconsin-Madison, where he is now fitness area coordinator. Dr. Bahrke is a fitness instructor and a strength and conditioning specialist certified by the National Strength and Conditioning Association. He is also included in the U.S. Olympic Committee Sports Psychology Registry.

David L. Bennell has over 7 years of experience as a drug prevention educator, with special emphasis on substance abuse prevention and student-athletes. He has a master's degree in health education from The Pennsylvania State University, where he helped pilot a national model drug prevention program for student-athletes. David is a training and development specialist for the Microsoft Corporation in Redmond, Washington.

Kirk J. Brower received his BA in psychobiology from the University of California, Los Angeles, and his MD from the University of California, Irvine. After completing his residency in psychiatry at UCLA in 1985, Dr. Brower joined the faculty at the University of Michigan in Ann Arbor, where he is currently an assistant professor of psychiatry. He is also executive director of the Chelsea Arbor Treatment Center, which is devoted to the treatment and research of substance abuse problems.

W.E. Buckley, PhD, is an associate professor in the Departments of Exercise and Sport Science and Health Education at The Pennsylvania State University. Dr. Buckley has been an athletic trainer at West Chester University and The Pennsylvania State University. He is a past chairperson of the Athletic Trainer Advisory Committee for Pennsylvania's Board of Physical Therapy Examiners. Dr. Buckley's research interests include sport injury rehabilitation, epidemiology, and substance abuse in sport.

Stephen P. Courson attended the University of South Carolina, where he was a tricaptain of the football team in 1976. He was drafted by the Pittsburgh Steelers in 1977 and was a member of the 1978 and 1979 Super Bowl championship teams. Mr. Courson was one of the first players to openly acknowledge his steroid use and the predicament in sports while still an active player (he did so in *Sports Illustrated* in 1985). He is now involved with Charles Yesalis in research and lectures to high schools, colleges, and civic groups about performance-enhancing drug use in sport and society. He has released his own book dealing with drugs in sport (*False Glory*, Longmeadow Press, 1991).

Jim Ferstle is a freelance writer who specializes in participatory sports, sports medicine, and education. He is a staff writer and running columnist for the St. Paul (Minnesota) *Pioneer Press*. Ferstle's award-winning reporting on drugs and sports for the *Pioneer Press* and other publications has brought him notoriety as an expert in the field. He was invited to lecture on anabolic steroids to medical students at the University of Minnesota in the fall of 1992. He also spent a year in London (fall of 1992 to fall of 1993) reporting from Europe on the sport and science scene.

Karl E. Friedl, PhD, is a research physiologist in the Occupational Physiology Division of the U.S. Army Research Institute of Environmental Medicine in Natick, Massachusetts. He is also a major in the U.S. Army. Dr. Friedl received his PhD in physiology from the University of California, Santa Barbara in 1984 and did postdoctoral studies in the physiology of androgen-binding proteins.

R. Craig Kammerer, PhD, is a senior research scientist at XenoBiotic Laboratories in Princeton, New Jersey. Dr. Kammerer has been assistant professor of pharmacology (1978-1987) at the UCLA School of Medicine and was the founding associate director of the Paul Ziffren Olympic Analytical Lab (1982-1987). This first IOC-accredited lab in the USA performed drug testing for the 23rd Summer Olympics in Los Angeles in 1984.

Charles D. Kochakian received his PhD in physiological chemistry in 1936 from the University of Rochester. A pioneer in the research of anabolic-androgenic steroids, Dr. Kochakian discovered the anabolic action of a male hormone extract of human urine, determined the sites of protein synthesis, and delineated the mechanism of action of testosterone on protein synthesis. Today he is a professor emeritus of the University of Alabama at Birmingham.

John Lombardo earned his MD from The Ohio State University, Columbus, where he is professor and chairman of the Department of Family Medicine. Dr. Lombardo also is medical director of the OSU Sports Medicine Center, team physician for the OSU athletic teams, and drug advisor to the NFL. He was head physician for the 1988 U.S. Winter Olympic Team in Calgary and has been team physician for the Cleveland Cavaliers and consultant to the Cleveland Browns. Dr. Lombardo is president of the American Medical Society for Sports Medicine.

Richard H. Strauss, MD, is a professor of preventive medicine and internal medicine at The Ohio State University and a team physician for their athletic department. He is also editor-in-chief of *The Physician and Sportsmedicine*. Dr. Strauss has done considerable research on anabolic-androgenic steroids and their use among athletes, including use by women.

Judith R. Vicary, PhD, is an associate professor of health education in the College of Health and Human Development, The Pennsylvania State University, and director of the Center for Worksite Health Enhancement. She has been a NIDA postdoctoral research fellow and is the principal investigator for a 7-year longitudinal study of adolescent development, including substance use. Dr. Vicary also directs a 5-year demonstration project, funded by the Office of Substance Abuse Prevention, to reduce the use of alcohol, tobacco, and other drugs among rural disadvantaged women.

James Wright holds a bachelor's degree in biology from Fairleigh Dickenson University and a doctoral degree in zoology from Mississippi State University. He has been an NIH postdoctoral fellow at the Institute of Environmental Stress, University of California, Santa Barbara. Wright served in the USMC and later in the U.S. Army, for which he was a research team leader and chief of the Muscle Strength Section at the U.S. Army Research Institute of Environmental Medicine (1977-1982). From 1985 to 1988 he was chief of the Exercise Science Branch at the U.S. Army Physical Fitness School and Liaison of the Office of the (Army) Surgeon General to that organization. Dr. Wright is currently an associate editor and technical advisor for Weider Health and Fitness in Los Angeles.

Preface

No one is guilty of steroid use except the other guy, the other team or the other school—what a laugh.

CHARLES YESALIS, SR.
Chicago Golden Gloves Team 1934
University of Illinois Basketball and Track 1935-36

The use of performance-enhancing drugs by athletes, most notably anabolic steroids, is likely the greatest problem facing sport today. Hardly a
week goes by that another revelation of drug use by high school, collegiate,
professional, or Olympic-level athletes is not highlighted in the news.
Professor Willdor Hollmann, head of the Cologne Institute for Sports
Medicine and Circulatory Research, said in 1985, "Never again, not even
in the remote future will we see a type of high performance sport without
doping problems" (Hoberman, 1987, p. 321). Given the magnitude of this
problem, it is important that physicians, athletic trainers, nurses, physical
therapists, and other medical professionals who treat and counsel athletes
have a thorough knowledge of performance-enhancing drugs.

For some time there has been a lack of trust and communication between
members of the athletic community and the scientific and medical communities regarding anabolic steroids and other drugs. This, in part, is a
function of a poor understanding by clinicians and researchers of the
motivations of athletes, and vice versa. The medical community has lost
much credibility as a result of repeated denials that anabolic steroids
enhance performance (American College of Sports Medicine [ASCM],
1977; Ryan, 1981). Until recently, physicians and scientists dogmatically
reported that any weight an athlete gains while taking steroids is mainly
the result of fluid retention and that any strength gain is largely psychological (a placebo effect). Furthermore, some members of the sports medicine
community have, with the best of intentions, adopted an overly aggressive
educational strategy and have used strong, but often unfounded, pro-
nouncements regarding the adverse health effects of anabolic steroids.
Athletes, on the other hand, simply have not witnessed long-time steroid
users "dropping like flies." This credibility gap has been exacerbated
by the apparent contradiction between these warnings of dire health
consequences and the 10-center worldwide trial sponsored by the World
Health Organization to test the efficacy of anabolic steroids as a male
contraceptive (World Health Organization Task Force on Methods for the
Regulation of Male Fertility, 1990). To help close this gap, our book seeks
to provide the reader with a comprehensive, accurate, and objective discussion of anabolic steroid use in sport.

The contributors to this text have spent a number of years researching
anabolic steroids, and they represent backgrounds in several areas of
science and clinical medicine as well as journalism. Most were among a
small, select group invited to either the National Institute on Drug Abuse
Technical Review on Anabolic Steroid Abuse or the National Consensus
Meeting on Anabolic Steroids sponsored by the National Collegiate Athletic Association, the U.S. Olympic Committee, and the Amateur Athletic

Foundation. Both these meetings, held in 1989, were milestones in that they helped focus the attention of the government, the sports medicine community, and sport federations on the magnitude of this problem. Many of the authors also have actively assisted the federal government and state governments as well as national sport federations in dealing with drug use in athletics. The authors have collaborated on this book to attempt to answer, at least in part, the following questions about anabolic steroids.

- What are anabolic steroids?
- Who uses anabolic steroids?
- Do anabolic steroids enhance physical capacities?
- How do anabolic steroids work?
- How do anabolic steroids affect physical and psychological health?
- What alternatives do we have as a society in dealing with this problem?

To best answer these questions, this book is divided into three parts. Part I, "History and Incidence of Use," contains four chapters that explain the chemical development of anabolic steroids and trace the progression of anabolic steroid use by athletes. Physical and psychological effects of these drugs as well as approaches to assessment and treatment are discussed in Part II, "Effects, Dependence, and Treatment Issues." The contributors to Part III, "Testing and Societal Alternatives," explain the origins, history, and problems of testing for anabolic steroids and pose some thought-provoking solutions to anabolic steroid use.

By providing our perspectives on these issues, we trust that this text will help clinicians and health educators better provide potential or current anabolic steroid users with the best information available with which to make informed judgments. Furthermore, we hope that this book will give health professionals a better understanding of anabolic steroid use in sport and will help them solve this societal problem.

References

American College of Sports Medicine. (1977). Position statement on the use and abuse of anabolic-androgenic steroids in sports. *Medicine and Science in Sports and Exercise*, **9**, 11-13.

Hoberman, J.M. (1987). Sport and the technological image of man. In W.J. Morgan & K.V. Meier (Eds.), *Philosophic inquiry in sport* (pp. 319-327). Champaign, IL: Human Kinetics.

Ryan, A. (1981). Anabolic steroids are fool's gold. *Federation Proceedings*, **40**, 2682-2688.

World Health Organization Task Force on Methods for the Regulation of Male Fertility. (1990). Contraceptive efficacy of testosterone-induced azospermia in normal men. *Lancet*, **336**, 955-959.

Credits

Chapter 1

Portions of this chapter are reprinted from "The Evolution From 'the Male Hormone' to Anabolic-Androgenic Steroids" by C.D. Kochakian, 1988, *Alabama Journal of Medical Sciences*, **25**(1), pp. 96-102. Reprinted by permission of the University of Alabama School of Medicine. The journal article is an abbreviated version of the November 1986 History of Medicine Seminar from the Reynolds Historical Library Lecture Series. The complete lecture was recorded on videotape and is available with the original manuscript from the Reynolds Library, University of Alabama at Birmingham. The lecture was also presented at the Panel on Steroid Abuse, National Institute of Drug Abuse, March 1989 (Kochakian, 1990a) and an abbreviated version has been published in *Trends in Biochemical Sciences*, 1986, **11**, pp. 399-400.

Figure 1.1 is from "New Experiments on Ovariotomy and the Problem of Sex Inversion in the Fowl" by L.V. Domm, 1927, *Journal of Experimental Zoology*, **48**(1), p. 151. Copyright © 1927. Reprinted by permission of Wiley-Liss, a division of John Wiley and Sons, Inc.

Figures 1.2 and 1.3 are from *Steroids* (pp. 505, 514) by L.F. Fieser and M. Fieser, 1959, New York: Reinhold. Copyright 1959 by Reinhold Publishing Corporation.

Figure 1.5 is from "Influence of Several C-19 Steroids on the Growth of Individual Muscles of the Guinea Pig" by C.D. Kochakian and C. Tillotson, 1957, *Endocrinology*, **60**, pp. 607-618. Reprinted by permission of the Endocrine Society.

Table 1.2 is from "Evaluation of the Protein Anabolic Properties of Certain Orally Active Anabolic Agents Based on Nitrogen Balance Studies in Rats" by A. Arnold, G.O. Potts, and A.L. Beyler, 1963, *Endocrinology*, **72**, pp. 408-417. Used by the permission of the Endocrine Society.

Table 1.3 is from "Anabolic Steroids in Clinical Medicine" by G.W. Liddle and H.A. Burke, Jr., 1960, *Helvetica Medica Acta*, **27**, p. 14. Reprinted by permission of Schwabe & Co. AG.

Chapter 3

Portions of this chapter are from "Athletes' Projections of Anabolic Steroid Use" by C.E. Yesalis, W.E. Buckley, W.A. Anderson, M.Q. Wang, J.A. Norwig, G. Ott, J.C. Puffer, and R.H. Strauss, 1990, *Clinical Sports Medicine*, **2**, pp. 155-171 and from "Anabolic-Androgenic Steroids: A Synthesis of Existing Data and Recommendations for Future Research" by C.E. Yesalis, J.E. Wright, & J.A. Lombardo, 1989, *Clinical Sports Medicine*, **1**, pp. 109-134. Copyright 1990, 1989 by Chapman & Hall Ltd. Reprinted by permission.

Tables 3.1-3.3 and 3.5 are from "Anabolic-Androgenic Steroids: A Synthesis of Existing Data and Recommendations for Future Research" by C.E. Yesalis, J.E. Wright, and J.A. Lombardo, 1989, *Clinical Sports Medicine*, **1**, pp. 111, 113, 114, and 116. Copyright 1989 by Chapman & Hall Ltd. Reprinted by permission.

Table 3.4 is from "Athletes' Projections of Anabolic Steroid Use" by C.E. Yesalis, W.E. Buckley, W.A. Anderson, M.Q. Wang, J.A. Norwig, G. Ott, J.C. Puffer, and R.H. Strauss, 1990, *Clinical Sports Medicine*, **2**, p. 168. Copyright 1990 by Chapman & Hall Ltd. Reprinted by permission.

Chapter 4, Tables 4.1-4.4, and Figures 4.1-4.3

Portions of this chapter (including the tables and figures) are from "Estimated Prevalence of Anabolic Steroid Use Among Male High School Seniors" by W.E. Buckley, C.E. Yesalis, K.E. Friedl, W.A. Anderson, A.L. Streit, and J.E. Wright, 1988, *Journal of the American Medical Association*, **260**(23), pp. 3441-3445. Copyright 1988, American Medical Association. Reprinted by permission.

Chapter 5

Portions of this chapter are from John A. Lombardo et al., "Anabolic/Androgenic Steroids and Growth Hormone" in David R. Lamb and Melvin H. Williams, Eds., *Perspectives in Exercise Science and Sports Medicine, Volume 4: Ergogenics—Enhancement of Performance in Exercise and Sport*. Copyright © 1991 Wm. C. Brown Communications, Inc., Dubuque, Iowa. All rights reserved. Reprinted by permission.

Chapter 5 list on page 90 is from "Stimulants" by J.A. Lombardo. In *Drugs & Performance in Sports* by R.H. Strauss (Ed.), 1987, Philadelphia: Saunders. Copyright 1987 by W.B. Saunders Company. Used by permission.

Table 5.2 is from John A. Lombardo et al., "Anabolic/Androgenic Steroids and Growth Hormone" in David R. Lamb and Melvin H. Williams, Eds., *Perspectives in Exercise Science and Sports Medicine, Volume 4: Ergogenics—Enhancement of Performance in Exercise and Sport*. Copyright © 1991 Wm. C. Brown Communications, Inc., Dubuque, Iowa. All rights reserved. Reprinted by permission.

Table 5.3 is from "Anabolic-Androgenic Steroids: A Synthesis of Existing Data and Recommendations for Future Research" by C.E. Yesalis, J.E. Wright, and J.A. Lombardo, 1989, *Clinical Sports Medicine*, **1**, p. 120. Copyright 1989 by Chapman & Hall Ltd. Reprinted by permission.

Tables 7.2-7.4 are from "Anabolic Steroid Use and Perceived Effects in Ten Weight-Trained Women Athletes" by R.H. Strauss, M.T. Liggett, and R.R. Lanese, 1985, *Journal of the American Medical Association*, **253**, pp. 2871-2873. Copyright 1985, American Medical Association. Adapted by permission.

Figures 7.1 and 7.2 are from "Endrocrine Effects in Women Weight Lifters Self-Administering Testosterone and Anabolic Steroids" by W.B. Malarkey, R.H. Strauss, D.J. Leizmen, M.T. Liggett, and L.M. Demers, 1991, *American Journal of Obstetrics and Gynecology*, **165**, pp. 1385-1390. Reprinted by permission of Mosby-Year Book, Inc.

Chapter 8

This chapter is adapted from "Psychological and Behavioural Effects of Endogenous Testosterone Levels and Anabolic-Androgenic Steroids Among Males: A Review" by M.S. Bahrke, C.E. Yesalis, and J.E. Wright, 1990, *Sports Medicine*, **10**(5), pp. 303-337. Copyright 1990 by Adis Press Ltd. Adapted by Permission.

Tables 9.1 and 9.2 are from "Symptoms and Correlates of Anabolic-Androgenic Steroid Dependence" by K.J. Brower, F.C. Blow, J.P. Young, and E.M. Hill, 1991, *British Journal of Addiction*, **86**, p. 763. Used by permission of Carfax Publishing Company.

Chapter 10

Portions of this chapter (including all the tables) are from "Anabolic Steroid Use: Indications of Habituation Among Adolescents" by C.E. Yesalis, A.L. Streit, J.R. Vicary, K.E. Friedl, D. Brannon, and W. Buckley, 1989, *Drug Education*, **19**(2), pp. 103-116. Published by Baywood Publishing Co., Inc. Copyright © 1989, Baywood Publishing Co., Inc. Reprinted by permission.

Chapter 11

Portions of this chapter and Table 11.1 are from "Withdrawal From Anabolic Steroids" by K.J. Brower. In *Current Therapy in Endocrinology and Metabolism* (4th ed., pp. 259-264) by C.W. Bardin, 1991, Philadelphia: Decker. Copyright 1991 by B.C. Decker. Used by permission.

Introduction

> *The pill, capsule, vial and needle have become fixtures of the locker room as athletes increasingly turn to drugs in the hope of improving performances. This trend ... poses a major threat to U.S. sport even though the Establishment either ignores or hushes up the issue.*
>
> BILL GILBERT
> *Sports Illustrated*, June–July, 1969

This introduction will provide the reader with a foundation for the discussion of anabolic steroids as well as develop a conceptual framework in which to place the chapters that follow. The introduction will define the term *anabolic-androgenic steroids* and will examine the reasons and methods for the use of steroids in sport and exercise. The use of drugs in sport as well as our societal concern for and knowledge of this issue will be placed in an historical context, and the underlying philosophical basis for our concern with this matter will be discussed.

Definition of Terms

Anabolic-androgenic steroids are synthetic derivatives of testosterone (see chapter 1). Testosterone, the natural male hormone that is produced primarily by the testes in men, is responsible for the androgenic (masculinizing) and anabolic (tissue-building) effects noted during male adolescence and adulthood. Androgenic effects are those that relate to the growth of the male reproductive tract or to the development of secondary sexual characteristics in men. In the pubertal male, these are increases in the length and diameter of the penis, development of the prostate and scrotum, and the appearance of the pubic, axillary, and facial hair. Anabolic effects are the changes that occur in the somatic and non–reproductive tract tissue; these include an acceleration of linear growth that appears before bony epiphyseal closure, enlargement of the larynx, thickening of the vocal cords, development of libido and sexual potentia, and an increase in muscle bulk and strength as well as a decrease in body fat.

Why and How Athletes Use Anabolic Steroids

The goals of individuals who use anabolic steroids depend upon the activities in which they participate. Bodybuilders desire more lean mass and less body fat. Weight lifters, both power and Olympic, desire to lift the maximum amount of weight possible. Field athletes want to put the shot or throw the hammer, discus, or javelin farther than competitors or record holders. Swimmers and runners hope to perform their frequent, high-intensity, long-duration workouts without physical breakdown. Football players want to increase their lean body mass and strength so that they can be successful at the high school, college, or professional level. Another group of users of anabolic steroids simply wants to look good, which currently means big and muscular.

Anabolic steroids have traditionally been taken in *cycles*, which are episodes of use lasting 6 to 12 weeks or more (Phillips, 1990). However, there are athletes, such as some power lifters, who use the drugs on a relatively continuous basis and increase their doses at certain times of the year, for example, to prepare for a competition (Duchaine, 1989). Often athletes will take more than one steroid at a time; this is referred to as *stacking*. The purported rationale for stacking is that it allows the user to activate more receptor sites than if only one steroid is used, or that the user can achieve a synergistic effect with certain combinations of steroids (Duchaine, 1989; Hatfield, 1982; Phillips, 1990). In order to avoid *plateauing* (developing a tolerance to a particular anabolic steroid), some users stagger their drugs and will take the steroids in an overlapping pattern or will stop taking one drug and start another—this does not necessarily mean that only one drug is taken at a time (Duchaine, 1989; Hatfield, 1982; Phillips, 1990). Often steroid users will *pyramid* their dosing patterns such that users move from low daily doses at the beginning of the cycle to higher doses and then taper their doses down toward the end of the cycle (Wright, 1982). In addition, the athlete may use a number of other drugs concurrently with anabolic steroids to further enhance physical capacities or to counteract the common side effects of steroids. These drugs include stimulants, diuretics, antiestrogens, human chorionic gonadotropin (HCG), human growth hormone (hGH), antiacneiform medications, as well as anti-inflammatories (Di Pasquale, 1984). This polypharmacy is termed an *array* (Duchaine, 1989).

Athletes primarily use the oral and intramuscular forms of anabolic steroids, and needle sharing has been reported, albeit infrequently (Yesalis, Wright, & Lombardo, 1989). More recently, it has been rumored that some elite athletes have begun using testosterone via transdermal patches, usually applied to the scrotum, and nasal sprays (Dickman, 1991) as potential means of circumventing drug tests (see chapter 13).

The dose of anabolic steroids depends on the sport as well as the particular needs of the athlete. Endurance athletes use steroids primarily for their alleged catabolism-blocking effects (Yesalis et al., 1989) and employ doses at or slightly below physiologic replacement levels, that is, about 7 mg per day (Yen & Jaffee, 1978). (Because the bioequivalence of various forms and types of anabolic steroids has not been established, the estimates of dosages used by athletes relative to physiologic replacement levels are approximate.) Although sprinters desire similar results, the strength and power requirements of their activity result in doses that are approximately one and one-half to more than double replacement levels (Francis, 1990). Participants in the traditional strength sports, seeking to "bulk up," have generally used amounts that exceed physiologic levels by 10 to 100 times or more (Kerr, 1982; Wright, 1982). Dosing patterns will also vary among athletes within a particular sport based on each athlete's training goals and response to the drugs and the biological activity of different anabolic steroids (Di Pasquale, 1984; Kerr, 1982; Kochakian, 1990; Wright, 1982). Women, regardless of sport, are thought to generally use lower doses of anabolic steroids than males (see chapter 7).

Sources of Anabolic Steroids

The majority of individuals who use anabolic steroids to enhance athletic performance and physical appearance obtain the drugs from the illicit market (Yesalis, Anderson, Buckley, & Wright, 1990). Black-market steroids come from three sources, which have roughly equal shares of the market, according to the Interagency Task Force on Anabolic Steroids (1991). One-third of the drugs are manufactured, legally or illegally, outside the United States and smuggled into this country; one-third are manufactured in this country by licensed pharmaceutical companies and diverted into the black market by the producer, distributor, pharmacist, veterinarian, or physician; and one-third come from clandestine laboratories. A minority of illicit users, probably less than 10%, obtain anabolic steroids by prescription. Because some of these drugs are counterfeit, the actual doses taken by illicit users are difficult to determine (Interagency Task Force on Anabolic Steroids, 1991). Moreover, some of the drugs taken are intended for veterinary use (Duchaine, 1989), so the equivalent human doses are unknown.

Is Drug Use New?

The use of drugs to enhance physical performance has been a feature of athletic competition since the beginning of recorded history (Prokop, 1970; Strauss & Curry, 1987). The legendary Berserkers of Norse mythology used bufotenin for stimulating effects, whereas West Africans used Cola accuminita and Cola nitida for running competitions since ancient times (Prokop, 1970; Boje, 1939). The ancient Greeks ate hallucinogenic mushrooms as well as sesame seeds to enhance performance, and the gladiators in the Roman Colosseum used stimulants to overcome fatigue and injury (Wadler & Hainline, 1989). For centuries South American Indians have chewed coca leaves to increase endurance (Boje, 1939; Karpovich, 1941).

During the 19th century, performance-enhancing drug use among athletes was commonplace. Swimmers, distance runners, sprinters, and cyclists used drugs such as caffeine, alcohol, nitroglycerine, digitalis, cocaine, strychnine, ether, opium, and heroin to get an edge over their opponents (Boje, 1939; Hoberman, in press; Prokop, 1970). Indeed the first fatality attributed to a performance-enhancing drug was that of an English cyclist who overdosed on tri-methyl during a race between Bordeaux and Paris in 1886 (Prokop, 1970). In 1939, in a paper entiteld "Doping," Boje stated,

> There can be no doubt that stimulants are to-day widely used by athletes participating in competitions; the record-breaking craze and the desire to satisfy an exacting public play a more and more prominent role, and take higher rank than the health of the competitors itself. (p. 439)

Today athletes employ a wide variety of drugs other than anabolic steroids to enhance performance; these include human growth hormone (hGH), erythropoietin, thyroid hormone, insulin, human chorionic gonadotropin (HCG), gonadotropin-releasing hormone, clenbuterol, L-dopa, gamma hydroxy butyrate (GHB), and chromium picolinate. Currently over 100 substances are banned by the International Olympic Committee, including over 17 anabolic steroids and related compounds.

Is Concern Over Drug Use New?

Prokop (1970) wrote that by the early 1930s the word *doping* had already been incorporated into our language, and not only had the medical aspects of drug use in sport been discussed but the moral and ethical aspects as well. In 1924 a German physician, Dr. Willner, wrote,

> At competitions we want to measure physical performances, not test the effects of drugs. . . . In my view, there is nothing more reprehensible than using pharmacological substances in an attempt to improve one's performances in competition with others who bring to the sporting encounter only that fitness that they have achieved through training. (Hoberman, in press)

In the same year, the German Association of Physicians for the Promotion of Physical Culture condemned doping on both medical and ethical grounds. Boje (1939) wrote that in regard to doping "the ethical and medical aspects are so intermingled that the problem as a whole becomes most confused" (p. 440).

ANABOLIC STEROIDS IN SPORT AND EXERCISE

Charles E. Yesalis, ScD
The Pennsylvania State University

Editor

Human Kinetics Publishers

Why Are We Concerned?

The most obvious reason we are concerned about anabolic steroid use in sport is that it is cheating—the use of these drugs violates the rules of virtually every sport federation (Wadler & Hainline, 1989). A more important question, however, is, Why have sport federations outlawed the use of these drugs?

Our concern over drug use in sport is generally founded in one or more of the following moral and ethical issues:

- The athlete may suffer physical or psychological harm as a result of drug use (Brown, 1984; Karpovich, 1941; Murray, 1983; Simon, 1984).
- The use of drugs by one athlete may coerce another athlete to use drugs to maintain parity (Murray, 1983; Simon, 1984).
- The use of drugs in sport is unnatural in that any resulting success is due to external factors (Murray, 1983).
- The athlete who uses drugs has an unfair advantage over athletes who do not use them (Gardner, 1989).

Although on its surface each argument has an intuitive appeal, each holds inconsistencies.

Physical Harm

Although protecting the health of participants by banning drugs is admirable, one must keep in mind that a number of sports are an inherent threat to life and limb, such as boxing, football, and auto racing. Moreover, due to the fervor of competition as well as the intensity, frequency, and duration of training, it is difficult to imagine an elite athlete in any sport who has not experienced some level of sport-related injury.

The rationale of banning drugs to protect the health of athletes assumes that performance-enhancing drugs are harmful under all circumstances. In the case of anabolic steroids, this assumption does not appear to hold. Anabolic steroids are approved for use in certain medical conditions (see chapter 1) at doses that approximate those currently used by a number of sprint and endurance athletes. Furthermore, the use of anabolic steroids in male contraception trials argues that some steroids can be used safely at moderate doses at least in the short term (World Health Organization Task Force on Methods for the Regulation of Male Fertility, 1990). The health effects of anabolic steroids will be discussed at length in chapter 6.

Coercion of Athletes

Some have argued that at the elite level of certain sports, namely weight lifting, field events in track, bodybuilding, and perhaps the line positions in football, an athlete either uses steroids or will not be able to compete effectively (Committee on the Judiciary, United States Senate, 1973 & 1989; Dubin, 1990; Francis, 1990; Wade, 1972; Yesalis et al., 1988). If this is true, potential competitors are coerced into using these drugs or "resign themselves to either accepting a competitive disadvantage or leaving the endeavor entirely" (Murray, 1983, p. 27). Although this circumstance is unfortunate, the final decision to use steroids or participate in the sport still lies with the athlete. Heavy weight training, a basic requirement of most strength and power sports, is itself a health risk that athletes are pressured to endure. Furthermore, this ethical dilemma is not peculiar to sport. If a scientist wishes to do laboratory research on virulent strains of viruses or bacteria, he or she must accept certain risks; the only way to completely avoid such risks is to not participate in this type of research.

Success Due to External Factors

Ideally, superior performance in sport should be a function of factors internal to the athlete, such as genetic endowment, intelligence, motivation, courage, and dedication. Thus, it is argued that drugs, in this instance anabolic steroids, are an external factor and therefore unnatural (Simon, 1984). Anabolic steroids are, however, a derivative of a hormone that is endogenous to the human body; athletes who use steroids are supplementing what is already there. Moreover, is there a difference between athletes' using anabolic steroids and their using vitamins, aspirin, amino acids, or corticosteroids, all of which are allowed by most sport governing bodies? The use of fiberglass poles, synthetic track surfaces, lifting suits, and high-tech tennis rackets raises similar questions of unnaturalness.

Unfair Advantage

The contention that anabolic steroids grant the user an unfair advantage is interesting in that the use of these drugs was banned at least 9 years before the sports medicine community acknowledged that steroids could enhance performance (American College of Sports Medicine, 1977, 1984; Wadler & Hainline, 1989). There is little or no doubt, however, among athletes that the use of steroids offers a competitive edge. Athletes who have access to elite coaches, the most sophisticated equipment, the latest training techniques, and the most knowledgeable sport scientists also have significant advantages over those who cannot avail themselves of such luxuries. Perhaps as Gardner (1989) pointed out,

> What renders a substance-gained advantage unacceptable, and what we may be ultimately objecting to, is not that an advantage is gained over other athletes but that one is gained over the sport itself—either its intended purpose or its conceived obstacles. (p. 68)

Once again the distinctions are unclear. Although corked bats, high-pressure golf balls, and swim fins are not allowed in their respective sports, fiberglass poles, ultralight racing bicycles, and compound bows are.

Moral and Philosophical Concerns

In summary, none of the traditional ethical arguments for banning the use of anabolic steroids in sport is without limitations. Perhaps the most compelling argument against steroid (or any drug) use in sport is that it is morally wrong because it reduces sport to competition between biochemical machines; "it dehumanizes by not respecting the status of athletes as persons" (Fraleigh, 1984, p. 25). When high jumpers take anabolic steroids and other performance-enhancing drugs, the competition is not decided by who has best developed his or her skill but whose body has taken the most effective drugs at the proper time at the most productive dosage.

Simon (1984) concluded

> It is of course true that the choice to develop one's capacity through drugs is a choice a person might make. Doesn't respect for persons require that we respect the choice to use performance enhancers as much as any other? The difficulty, I suggest, is the effect that such a choice has on the process of athletic competition itself. The use of performance-enhancing drugs in sports restricts the area in which we can be respected as persons. Although individual athletes certainly can make such a choice, there is a justification inherent in the nature of good competition for prohibiting participation by those who make such a decision. Accordingly, the use of performance-enhancing drugs should be prohibited in the name of the value of respect for persons itself. (p. 13)

Sport should be a quest for personal excellence through competition, as well as a source of fun, enjoyment, and camaraderie. Drugs are unnecessary to achieve these ends. If the primary objective of participation in sport, however, is to achieve victory over an opponent, the use of drugs to achieve that end becomes an increasingly rational behavior.

Has Steroid Use Been a Secret?

Some might think that until recently the dimensions of the problem of steroid use in sport were the privileged information of a few insiders. This is not true. In 1969, *Sports Illustrated* (Gilbert, 1969a, 1969b, 1969c) published a three-part series on drug use that named athletes and sports and detailed the magnitude of the issue; between 1971 and 1972 *Science* and the *New York Times Magazine* published similar articles (Wade, 1972; Scott, 1971). As a result of these and like revelations, the United States Senate Committee on the Judiciary held hearings in 1973 on drug use in sports (Committee on the Judiciary, United States Senate, 1973); no new laws resulted and public interest dwindled.

With the possible exception of a few comments made in the news media during the 1970s, such as comments related to the masculine appearances of some Eastern Bloc female athletes, little public attention was given to the use of performance-enhancing drugs until the 1983 Pan American Games in Caracas, Venezuela. During these games international attention was focused on 19 athletes (two from the United States) who tested positive for anabolic steroids and on a number of U.S. athletes who returned home prior to competition to, in the minds of many, avoid detection and sanctions. Three years later Brian Bosworth and 25 other college football players were suspended from postseason competition for anabolic steroid use. Once again, public interest appeared to subside, and it was not until the fall of 1988 that the issue was thrust once more into the spotlight when Ben Johnson was stripped of his gold medal at the Seoul Olympics. Since that time the media, governments, and sport federations have given significant attention to assessing the magnitude of the problem and identifying alternative solutions.

Why has it taken several decades to develop a sustained level of public and sport federation interest as well as government scrutiny? For one thing, the fact that high school students have been using anabolic steroids has only recently been given wide public exposure (Buckley et al., 1988). Another reason for the apparent intensification of activity on drug use in sport during the late 1980s was timing. Ironically, our society was confronted with the news of adolescent steroid use only 1 month after the Ben Johnson incident—all of this took place during a period of heightened concern over illicit drug use, especially among young people. The negative image of drug use and its potential deleterious effect on the marketing of collegiate, Olympic, and professional sport might explain, in part, the apparent lack of motivation of many sport officials in dealing with this problem during the prior 30 years.

Conclusion

In the past several thousand years, humans have tried numerous substances to enhance their performance. Anabolic steroids and a rapidly growing list of other drugs are merely the 20th century's contribution to this endeavor. Long before a world sport figure was stripped of his medal at the Seoul Olympics, concerned voices—most often unheeded—warned of the problem of drug use and other excesses in sport. Their concerns about drug use included the well-being of the athlete, coercion to cheat, unfair advantage, and excellence achieved through artificial means. In the end, however, the main effect of drug use in sport is to degrade athletic competition to a battle of biochemical machines.

References

American College of Sports Medicine. (1977). Position statement on the use and abuse of anabolic-androgenic steroids in sports. *Medicine and Science in Sports and Exercise*, **9**, 11-13.

American College of Sports Medicine. (1984). Position stand on the use of anabolic-androgenic steroids in sports. *Sports Medicine Bulletin*, **19**, 13-18.

Boje, O. (1939). Doping. *Bulletin of the Health Organization of the League of Nations*, **8**, 439-469.

Brown, W.M. (1984). Paternalism, drugs, and the nature of sport. *Journal of the Philosophy of Sport*, **XI**, 14-22.

Buckley, W.E., Yesalis, C.E., Friedl, K.E., Anderson, W., Streit, A., & Wright, J. (1988). Estimated prevalence of anabolic steroid use among male high school seniors. *Journal of the American Medical Association*, **260**(23), 3441-3445.

Committee on the Judiciary, United States Senate; Subcommittee to Investigate Juvenile Delinquency. (1973). *Proper and improper use of drugs by athletes*. Ninety-third Congress, first session, June 18 and July 12 and 13, 1973.

Committee on the Judiciary, United States Senate. (1989). *Steroids in amateur and professional sports—the medical and social costs of steroid abuse*. One hundred first Congress, first session, April 3, 1989, Newark, DE; May 9, 1989, Washington, DC.

Dickman, S. (1991). East Germany: Science in the disservice of the state. *Science*, **254**, 26-27.

Di Pasquale, M.G. (1984). *Drug use and detection in amateur sports.* Warkworth, ON: M.G.D. Press.

Dubin, C. (1990). *Commission of inquiry into the use of drugs and banned practices intended to increase athletic performance* (Catalog No. CP32-56/1990E, ISBN 0-660-13610-4). Ottawa, ON: Canadian Government Publishing Center.

Duchaine, D. (1989). *Underground steroid handbook II.* Venice, CA: HLR Technical Books.

Fraleigh, W.P. (1984). Performance-enhancing drugs in sport: The ethical issue. *Journal of the Philosophy of Sport*, **XI**, 23-29.

Francis, C. (1990). *Speed trap.* New York. St. Martin's Press.

Gardner, R. (1989). On performance-enhancing substances and the unfair advantage argument. *Journal of the Philosophy of Sport*, **XVI**, 59-73.

Gilbert, B. (1969a, June 23). Drugs in sport: Part 1. Problems in a turned-on world. *Sports Illustrated*, pp. 64-72.

Gilbert, B. (1969b, June 30). Drugs in sport: Part 2. Something extra on the ball. *Sports Illustrated*, pp. 30-42.

Gilbert, B. (1969c, July 7). Drugs in sport: Part 3. High time to make some rules. *Sports Illustrated*, pp. 30-35.

Hatfield, F. (1982). *Anabolic steroids: What kind and how many.* Venice, CA: Fitness System.

Hoberman, J. (in press). The early development of sports medicine in Germany. In J. Berryman & R. Park (Eds.), *Sport and exercise science: Essays in the history of sports medicine.* Champaign: University of Illinois Press.

Interagency Task Force on Anabolic Steroids. (1991, January). Washington, DC: U.S. Department of Health and Human Services, Public Health Service.

Karpovich, P.V. (1941). Ergogenic aids in work and sports. *Research Quarterly*, **12**(Suppl.), 432-450.

Kerr, R. (1982). *The practical use of anabolic steroids with athletes.* San Gabriel, CA: Kerr.

Kochakian, C.D. (1990). History of anabolic-androgenic steroids. In G. Linn & L. Erinoff (Eds.), *Anabolic steroid abuse* (NIDA Research Monograph No. 102). Rockville, MD: National Institute on Drug Abuse.

Murray, T.H. (1983). The coercive power of drugs in sports. *The Hastings Center Report*, **13**(24), 24-30.

Phillips, W. (1990). *Anabolic reference guide* (5th ed.). Golden, CO: Mile High.

Prokop, L. (1970). The struggle against doping and its history. *Journal of Sports Medicine and Physical Fitness*, **10**(1), 45-48.

Scott, J. (1971, October 17). It's not how you play the game, but what pill you take. *New York Times Magazine*.

Simon, R.L. (1984). Good competition and drug-enhanced performance. *Journal of the Philosophy of Sport*, **XI**, 6-13.

Strauss, R.H., & Curry, T.J. (1987). Magic, science and drugs. In R.H. Strauss (Ed.), *Drugs and performance in sports* (pp. 3-9). Philadelphia: Saunders.

Wade, N. (1972). Anabolic steroids: Doctors denounce them, but athletes aren't listening. *Science*, **176**, 1399-1403.

Wadler, G., & Hainline, B. (1989). *Drugs and the athlete*. Philadelphia: Davis.

World Health Organization Task Force on Methods for the Regulation of Male Fertility. (1990). Contraceptive efficacy of testosterone-induced azospermia in normal men. *The Lancet*, **336**, 955-959.

Wright, J. (1982). *Anabolic steroids and sport II*. Natick, MA: Sports Science Consultants.

Yen, S., & Jaffe, R. (1978). *Reproductive endocrinology*. Philadelphia: Saunders.

Yesalis, C.E., Herrick, R.T., Buckley, W.E., Friedl, K.E., Brannon, D., & Wright, J.E. (1988). Self-reported use of anabolic-androgenic steroids by elite power lifters. *The Physician and Sportsmedicine*, **16**, 91-100.

Yesalis, C.E., Wright, J.E., & Lombardo, J.A. (1989). Anabolic-androgenic steroids: A synthesis of existing data and recommendations for future research. *Clinical Sports Medicine*, **1**, 109-134.

Yesalis, C.E., Anderson, W.A., Buckley, W.E., & Wright, E. (1990). Incidence of the nonmedical use of anabolic-androgenic steroids. In G.C. Lin & L. Erinoff (Eds.), *Anabolic steroid abuse* (National Institute on Drug Abuse Research Monograph Series No. 102; DHHS Publication No. ADM90-1720; pp. 97-112). Rockville, MD: U.S. Department of Health and Human Services; Public Health Service; Alcohol, Drug Abuse, and Mental Health Administration.

PART I

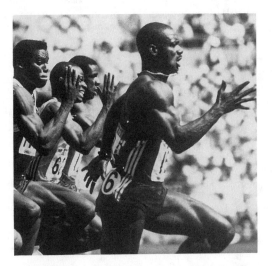

History and Incidence of Use

This part lays the groundwork for the study of anabolic steroids. Not only will you gain a detailed knowledge of the history of anabolic steroids and their use, but you will also read about the current level of use among students at the secondary school level and methodological problems associated with researching anabolic steroid use.

In chapter 1, Charles Kochakian provides a historical perspective of anabolic steroids. He discusses the loss of secondary male sex characteristics by castration, the family of male hormones termed *androgens*, the discovery of the male hormone testosterone, the discovery of the anabolic activity of testosterone, and the attempt to modify the testosterone molecule, resulting in anabolic-androgenic steroids. Kochakian also describes therapeutic and veterinary applications of anabolic steroids.

Whereas chapter 1 deals with the history of the development of anabolic steroids, chapter 2 details the history of anabolic steroid use, especially as this relates to use in sport and exercise settings. The authors describe the history of use among several categories of athletes, from Olympic level to high school. Of particular interest are factors mentioned that influenced the spread of steroid use from one class of athlete to another.

1

In chapter 3, Charles Yesalis critiques drug testing associated with sport competition as a method of assessing the level of steroid use. He also reviews the results of systematic surveys of anabolic steroid use given to adolescent and adult populations. He provides information gained from both of these assessment measures and discusses methodological problems related to these processes.

The data mentioned in chapter 3 along with anecdotal accounts from high school athletes, coaches, and athletic administrators suggesting widespread anabolic steroids use prompted a ground-breaking survey conducted in 1988. Chapter 4 presents the methods and results of this first nationwide survey of anabolic steroid use among the general adolescent male population. It also discusses possible methods of prevention.

CHAPTER 1

Anabolic-Androgenic Steroids: A Historical Perspective and Definition

Charles D. Kochakian

The more we understand how past discoveries have been made, the better we are able to plan for future discoveries.

W.I.B. BEVERIDGE
Frontiers in Comparative Medicine, 1972

Portions of this chapter are reprinted from Kochakian (1988) by permission; see credits page for more information.

In this chapter I will discuss the historical development and definition of anabolic steroids. I will also discuss the loss of the secondary male sex characteristics in fowls and men by castration, the discovery of the male hormone testosterone (the endocrine function of the testis), the family of male hormones termed *androgens*, the discovery of the anabolic activity of testosterone (the synthesis of new tissue), and the attempt to modify the testosterone molecule to produce a steroid with strong anabolic activity and no or very weak androgenic activity. These modified steroids became popularized as anabolic steroids, but they contain sufficient androgenic activity to produce virilization and have been classified along with testosterone as *anabolic-androgenic steroids*. Testosterone, in the form of several potent esters, and many of the modified steroids have been explored therapeutically in humans and in animals with surprising results; this research has explored the abilities of these drugs to correct a variety of conditions of protein deficiency and more recently to increase musculature and performance by athletes, race horses, and dogs.

Endocrine Function of the Testis

The scientific community did not recognize the endocrine function of the testis until almost 100 years after the initial demonstration by Berthold in 1849. Berthold's experiments and interpretation of the results clearly anticipated the fundamentals of endocrinology; 56 years later Starling (1905) named the blood-borne factors *hormones* (which means "to excite or arouse").

In this section I will describe the evolution and initiation of the concept that the testis produces a chemical substance that is secreted into the bloodstream and carried to the target tissues—the comb and wattles of the rooster and the accessory sex organs of the rat—to effect their growth and maintenance.

Castration and Secondary Male Characteristics

It has been known for centuries that castration of the male results in the loss of not only fertility but also the secondary male sex characteristics (Hoskins, 1941; Spencer, 1946). The Neolithic peoples of Asia Minor practiced castration as early as 4000 B.C. to domesticate animals for work and meat production (Spencer, 1946).

The practice of castration of humans probably originated in Babylonia about 2000 B.C., originally as a punitive measure (e.g., for adultery), and traveled to India by 1500 B.C., to Egypt by 1200 B.C., to China by 1122 B.C., and to other neighboring countries (Spencer, 1946). The practice flourished in the early days of the Eastern Roman Empire and was used by the early Christian Church for its priesthood and to retain the soprano voices of choirboys. Castration was forbidden at the Church Council of Nicea in A.D. 325. However, as late as the early 20th century religious cults (e.g., the Skoptz) continued the practice (Spencer, 1946). The Greeks and later the Romans did not accept the concept of castration probably because of their emphases on physical culture and the Olympic games (Spencer, 1946).

Early Primitive Attempts to Reverse Effects of Castration

Primitive people commonly ate organs of animals and even of humans to improve or cure the dysfunction of their respective organs. As early as 140 B.C.. Sucruta of India advocated the ingestion of testis tissue for the cure of impotence (Newerla, 1943). The endocrine function of the testis was speculated upon by Arataeus in about A.D. 150 and more vigorously by deBordeu in 1775. They proposed that each organ of the body produces a substance that is secreted into the blood to regulate bodily function. Although this concept touched upon the now-recognized function of the endocrine glands, it was mere speculation based on casual observation. However, early scientists made some progress in the knowledge of the anatomy and physiology of the testis. Aristotle (300 B.C.) described a clear conception of the effect of castration on the bird (capon). Furthermore, in the first half of the 19th century scientists recognized that the ductless glands are closely allied with the vascular system (Newerla, 1943).

In 1889, a respected French physician, Brown-Sequard, reported that aqueous extracts of animal testes injected into other animals (e.g., dogs) and even into himself produced improvements in general health, muscular strength, appetite, regulation of the intestinal tract, and mental faculties. Ironically, these uncontrolled studies and bold claims stimulated an increase in clinical endocrinology. Numerous similar reports soon followed and continued until the early 1920s. Surgeons developed lucrative practices by transplanting testes from animals (e.g., monkeys), and internists administered injections of aqueous and glycerol extracts of animal testes. It seemed that the fountain of youth had been discovered. But serious experimentation in reproduction, initiated in the 1920s (Parkes, 1966, 1985), caused scientists to become concerned with the blatant claims of rejuvenation. An international committee that was appointed to investigate concluded that claims of rejuvenation as a result of testis transplantation or injection of testicular extracts were unfounded (Parkes, 1985, 1988).

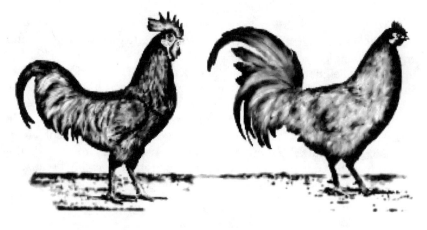

Figure 1.1   Effect of castration on the comb and wattles of the brown leghorn rooster. *Note.* Reprinted from Domm. (1927) by permission; see also Moore (1939).

The practice disappeared as scientists learned how to produce active extracts and then isolated, characterized, and synthesized the active substance.

Discovery of the Endocrine Function of the Testis

In spite of the early speculations, the general consensus as late as the middle of the 19th century was that the changes after castration were mediated through the nervous system. The first inkling as to the real regulation of these changes was provided in 1849 by Berthold, professor of medicine at Gottingen. In a simple and excellently designed experiment with only six roosters, he demonstrated that the well-known regression of the comb and wattles (see Figure 1.1) and changes in behavior, all of which occurred after castration, were prevented by the transplantation of the testis in the abdominal cavity. The transplants developed new blood supplies and maintained the roosters in the normal manner. Berthold correctly deduced that because the transplanted testis no longer had its nerve connections, it produced something that was secreted into the bloodstream and transported to the target tissues to regulate their growth and maintenance.

In the subsequent 60 years, Berthold's results were questioned. Others who attempted to repeat the transplantation experiments were unsuccessful except for Lode (1891, 1895), who did confirm Berthold's experiment but whose results were ignored. Pezard in 1911 successfully repeated the effects of castration in roosters and in 1912 fragmented the removed testes and deposited the fragments in the abdominal cavities of the castrated roosters (capons). The size of the combs and wattles of the capons were maintained.

Preparation of Active Extracts of Testis and Male Urine: Male Hormone

In the early 1920s, interest in the development of the male reproductive tract was accelerated. Many studies of laboratory rodents were conducted, and extracts of the testis were prepared that reversed the effects of castration (Moore, 1939). Regeneration—of the regressed accessory sex organ of the castrated rat (Moore, 1939; Moore & Gallagher, 1930), and the seminal vesicles of the castrated mouse (Voss, 1930)—was suggested as a method of assay.

In 1927, McGee reported that an alcohol extract of bull testicles stimulated the growth of the capon comb. Gallagher and Koch (1930) developed the stimulation of growth of the capon comb into a quantitative procedure and improved the extraction procedure to produce a highly purified and very active preparation (Gallagher & Koch, 1934b).

In the meantime Pezard and Caridroit in 1926 transplanted two fragments of the comb of a normal rooster to its back through an incision in the skin and found that the fragments were maintained (i.e., they did not regress). Another rooster was castrated, and 1 week later two fragments of the comb were transplanted to its back; both the comb in situ and the transplanted fragments exhibited the usual postcastration regression. The researchers deduced as had Berthold that the active principal was in the blood and that it acted directly on the comb. On the basis of this observation, Funk and Harrow in 1929 assumed that the active substance should be cleared by the kidney and appear in the urine. The researchers found that a crude concentrate of alcohol-treated male urine stimulated the growth of the capon comb. Acidification of the urine, followed by chloroform extraction, provided an oily active concentrate (Funk, Harrow, & Lejwa, 1930). Further purification and an increase in yield were effected by stronger acidification prior to chloroform extraction, followed by hydrolysis of the extract with sodium hydroxide solution (Funk & Harrow, 1930), which removed many impurities and also estrogens. Other investigators (Freud, deJongh, Laqueur, & Munch, 1930; Loewe & Voss, 1930) almost simultaneously developed similar extraction procedures. Thus, relatively simple methods for the assay and production of highly active concentrates of what was designated the "male hormone" became available.

Androgens: Multiplicity of Male Hormones

Androsterone, a substance with the ability to stimulate the growth of the capon comb, was isolated from human male urine and synthesized from cholesterol. This event was quickly followed by the isolation, synthesis, and chemical characterization of the biologically active principal in bull testes, testosterone, which was biologically more active and chemically slightly different from androsterone. The isolation of other chemically related and biologically active compounds from human male urine suggested that testosterone was metabolized in the body to several other related steroids. Appraisal of the testosterone molecule indicates that testosterone has the potential to be oxidized or reduced to approximately 600 related steroids. These steroids have been given the general name of androgens (*andro* = male; *gen* = to produce).

Isolation and Characterization of Androsterone

Butenandt (1931) succeeded in isolating 15 mg of a pure substance (Butenandt & Tscherning, 1934a) from an extract of 25,000 L of policemen's urine. Analysis of the urinary product (Butenandt & Tscherning, 1934b) indicated a hydroxyl and a ketone attached to a polycyclic nucleus like that of cholesterol; the researchers named this substance *androsterone* (*andro* = male, *ster* = sterol, *one* = ketone).

The final elucidation of the ring structure of cholesterol was in the process of being accomplished (see Fieser & Fieser, 1959). Ruzicka (1973), in the meantime, had become intrigued by the possible polycyclic structure of androsterone. Ruzicka, Goldberg, Meyer, Brunigger, and Eichenburg (1934) oxidized cholesterol and obtained the anticipated ketone. The free compound possessed only one-seventh the comb-growth-stimulating property of androsterone and was assumed to be a stereoisomer of androsterone. Ruzicka's group then immediately proceeded to convert cholesterol to androsterone and its three possible isomers (Figure 1.2). Thus, the chemical structure of androsterone and its relationship to cholesterol were established.

Synthesis, Isolation, and Characterization of Testosterone

The biological and chemical properties of the newly synthesized androsterone were compared with those of the testis extract; the testis extract was more active in the stimulation of growth of the seminal vesicles and prostate of the castrated rat and mouse (Freud et al., 1930), and it was labile to hot alkali (Gallagher & Koch, 1934a). The alkaline lability, based

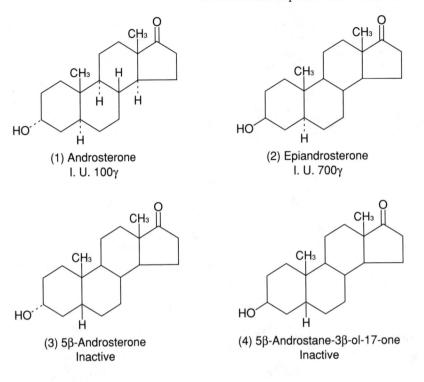

Figure 1.2 Androsterone and its three isomers. *Note.* Reprinted from Fieser & Fieser (1959); see credits page; see also Ruzicka et al. (1934).

on studies with progesterone, suggested the presence of an α, β-unsaturated ketone in the testis product (see Fieser & Fieser, 1959; Tausk, 1984). Both Ruzicka and Wettstein (1935a) and Butenandt and Kudszus (1935) immediately (in July 1935) reported the synthesis of androstenedione from cholesterol. The compound possessed the chemical lability of the testis extract and showed a substantial increase in biological activity, but it was not as biologically active as the testis extract. In August, Butenandt and Hanisch (1935) and Ruzicka and Wettstein (1935b) quickly converted the ketone at position 17 to a hydroxyl (Figure 1.3). This compound proved to have both the chemical and biological properties of the partially purified bull testis extract.

In May 1935, David of Laqueur's group in Amsterdam reported the isolation of a crystalline compound from bull testes (10 mg of 100 kg) that had the chemical and biological properties of the compound newly synthesized by the Butenandt and Ruzicka groups, and named it testosterone. Shortly thereafter, the Amsterdam group (David, Dingemanse, Freud, & Laqueur, 1935) reported that the chemical structure of their compound was identical with that of the recently synthesized compound.

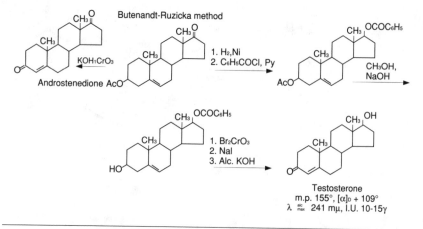

Figure 1.3   Synthesis of androstenedione and testosterone from cholesterol via dehydrepiandrosterone. *Note*. Reprinted from Fieser & Fieser (1959); see credits page.

Family of Related C$_{19}$-Steroids

It was becoming apparent that the body produces more than one compound with male hormonelike activity. Butenandt and Dannenbaum (1934) already had isolated dehydroandrosterone and a second compound from the male urine extract, an artifact (chlorodehydroandrosterone) of dehydroandrosterone formed during the hydrochloric acid hydrolysis of the urine. Furthermore, they indicated that there probably were several more related compounds present in the urine, which was amply confirmed over the subsequent years (Dorfman & Ungar, 1965). Thus, a family of compounds had been discovered, which was soon given the generic name *androgens*.

Testosterone has the potential to be converted by tissue enzymes to 27 compounds (Kochakian, 1959, 1990b). The polycyclic nucleus of each compound has nine potential sites for α- or β-hydroxylation and also potential hydroxylation of the angular methyls at C$_{18}$ and C$_{19}$. Thus it is possible for the tissues to produce at least another 540 compounds (Kochakian, 1990a, 1990b). Moreover, the unsaturated steroids may be converted to estrogens. Many of these compounds are already recognized (Kochakian, 1959; Kochakian & Arimasa, 1976).

In 1935, Ruzicka, Goldberg, and Rosenberg (see Fieser & Fieser, 1959) reported that the substitution of a methyl for the 17α-hydrogen yielded a highly effective oral compound, 17α-methyltestosterone, which was immediately accepted for clinical use. Testosterone in the early studies (Foss, 1939) appeared to be completely ineffective by oral administration, but later studies of mice (Kochakian, 1952) and humans (Johnsen, Bennett, & Jensen, 1974) demonstrated that testosterone was active by mouth if administered in sufficient quantity.

It was observed early (see Kochakian, 1938) that the addition of fatty acids or impurities from extracts enhanced the biological activity of a parenterally administered oil solution of testosterone. These studies (see Kochakian, 1938) suggested that esters of testosterone would prove effective. The acetates of testosterone and related compounds already were available; they had been prepared to establish the presence of hydroxyl in the molecule. On bioassay, the acetate of testosterone proved to be more effective and also to provide a more prolonged activity. The propionate was even more effective (see Kochakian, 1938) and became the standard compound for parenteral administration. The further prolongation of activity with the propionate prompted the synthesis of several other esters with even greater extension of activity that correlated with the length of the carbon chain of the carboxylic acid. The prolongation of biological activity has been extended as long as 4 months after the single injection of testosterone-trans-4n-butylcyclohexyl-carboxylate (Weinbauer, Marshall, & Nieschlag, 1986).

The introduction and recognition of 5α-dihydrotestosterone, 5α-dihydro-19-nor-testosterone, and 19-nortestosterone as effective agents were followed by the preparation of esters of these steroids. The esters are hydrolyzed by blood and/or tissue esterases to release the steroid for biological action.

Anabolic Activity

The discovery that testosterone stimulates the synthesis of new tissue opened many potential new uses for this steroid. I found that a male hormonelike extract from male urine stimulated a strong positive nitrogen balance in castrated dogs. As soon as androstenedione and testosterone were synthesized from cholesterol, these steroids were found also to produce a strong positive nitrogen effect in the castrated dogs. Shortly thereafter, testosterone propionate became commercially available and proved to produce an identical effect in eunuchoid men.

Nitrogen Balance in Dog and Man

The demonstration of male hormonelike activity in male urine stimulated many biological studies. Murlin, the discoverer of glucagon, was prompted to investigate whether this material also was responsible for the difference in basal metabolic rate (BMR) between males and females. He assigned two medical students in 1931 to conduct a pilot study as their class project. They found that an extract of medical student urine (similar to extracts studied by Funk, Harrow, & Lejwa, 1930) increased the BMR of a castrated dog. In the fall of 1933, I was appointed as a graduate assistant (Kochakian, 1984) to confirm and extend this exciting observation. In spite of repeated experiments on a similar extract at several dose levels, I was unable to confirm the increase in BMR. Thereupon, Murlin suggested the investigation of protein metabolism, a suggestion probably prompted by his earlier (1911) studies on nitrogen balance in pregnant dogs. The urine extract produced an immediate and strongly positive nitrogen balance in two castrated dogs. The results were reported in 1935 (Kochakian, 1935; Kochakian & Murlin, 1935) at the same time that androsterone, androstenedione, and testosterone were being characterized and synthesized. The experiments were immediately repeated with androstenedione (Kochakian & Murlin, 1936), which I synthesized from cholesterol by the method of the Butenandt and Ruzicka groups (see Figure 1.3), and testosterone and testosterone acetate (Kochakian, 1937), which had become commercially available, to give results identical with those of the urinary extract. Shortly thereafter, Kenyon, Sandiford, Bryan, Knowlton, and Koch (1938) reported identical results in eunuchoid men with the commercially available testosterone propionate. In addition to the retained nitrogen, the other elements (Na^+, K^+, Cl^-, H_2O, PO_4^{-3}) for the synthesis of new tissue were retained by the subjects in proportionate amounts.

The experiments involving the castrated dogs and the eunuchoid men clearly indicated that the secretion of the testis (testosterone) not only regulated the development of the secondary male characteristics and the accessory sex organs but also had a general anabolic effect. Subsequent experiments in rats, mice, guinea pigs, and hamsters demonstrated that testosterone influenced the synthesis of new tissue in practically every organ of the body. Thus testosterone is a general anabolic agent (Kochakian, 1975, 1976c).

Nitrogen Balance in Rats

Nitrogen balance studies in dogs proved to be too expensive and time-consuming. Therefore, these studies were extended to rats as one phase in the delineation of the nature and mechanism of the action of testosterone. The comparison of available natural androgens demonstrated testosterone propionate to be the most active; androsterone showed only a trace of activity (Kochakian, 1950, 1964). Testosterone was more active than androsterone but less active than testosterone propionate. The esterification enhanced and prolonged the activity. The various steroids produced a log/dose response.

An unexpected effect on the positive nitrogen balance and a simultaneous increase in body weight was revealed. Prolongation of the injections after 7 to 10 days resulted in a gradual return of the positive nitrogen balance to equilibrium and a cessation of the increase in body weight, followed by a gradual decrease to the initial level. This "wearing-off" effect could be reversed by increasing the dose of the steroid.

An identical pattern of response was reproduced with testosterone propionate in the normal male rat, the normal and ovariectomized female rat, the normal and castrated hypophysectomized male rat, the castrated-adrenalectomized rat, the surgically and thiouracil hypothyroid male rat, and the alloxan-diabetic rat (and the depancreatized dog). This indicated that the protein-synthesizing activity of testosterone and related steroids was not mediated through any of the other endocrine glands.

Partial Dissociation of Anabolic Activity From Androgenic Activity

The potential therapeutic usefulness of the protein-synthesizing property of testosterone in patients who exhibited a decrease in the formation of tissue was immediately recognized. The use of testosterone in such patients, however, was always accompanied with the virilizing effect, especially evident in women and children. The first indication that it might be possible to avoid this effect surfaced in experimentation on castrated mice, in the comparison of the differential effect of a number of natural steroids on the kidney weight as representative of the anabolic activity and on the prostates and seminal vesicles as representative of the androgenic activity. In general, the reduction of the polar groups of testosterone resulted in a decrease in androgenic activity without decreasing the weight of the kidney. A comparable relationship was obtained in a comparison of the response of the sensitive muscles of the castrated male guinea pig. A comparison of the response of the levator ani muscle with that of the prostate or seminal vesicles of the castrated rat was suggested as a simple and inexpensive screening assay to find a chemically modified testosterone which would have no or weak androgenic activity but have retained or enhanced activity of the muscle. Many modifications of testosterone were synthesized and exploited in clinical use as anabolic steroids. Unfortunately, the dissociation was never sufficient to prevent the residual virilizing activity from occurring.

Renotrophic/Androgenic Activity in Mice and Rats

The potential therapeutic value of the anabolic activity of testosterone and its commercial availability stimulated many investigations of diverse anabolic-deficient conditions (Landau, 1976; Reifenstein, 1942), including intensive studies in women with breast cancer. The clinical use, however, always presented the accompanying virilization, especially evident in women and children. A possible answer to this problem appeared imminent (Kochakian, 1942). As one aspect of my program to elucidate the nature and mechanism of the anabolic action, I decided to compare the abilities of a number of steroids to stimulate growth in the sensitive mouse kidney (anabolic effect) (Kochakian, 1977; Pfeiffer, Emmel, & Gardner, 1940; Selye, 1939) with their abilities to stimulate growth in the seminal vesicles and prostate (androgenic effect).

These studies indicated for the first time a possible separation of the stimulation of growth in two target tissues through a modification of the testosterone molecule. Reduction in the A-ring decreased the androgenic activity without significantly changing the renotrophic activity. The opposite effect was produced by oxidation of the 17-hydroxyl (Kochakian, 1944, 1946). I noted a similar response in the castrated rat (Kochakian, 1964). An even more striking dichotomous effect was produced by the oral administration of the mono-oxygenated steroid, 17α-methyl-5α-androstan-17β-ol (Kochakian, 1952). In 1961 another steroid without a 3-ketone (17α-ethylestrenol) demonstrated a favorable dissociation between its effect on the weight of the levator ani muscle and that of the prostate of the rat (see Potts, Arnold, & Beyler, 1976).

Myotrophic/Androgenic Activity in Guinea Pigs

Papanicolaou and Falk (1938) had reported that the temporal and the masseter muscles of the guinea pig were much larger in the male than in the female and that castration of the male resulted in female-sized muscles. Administration of testosterone propionate restored the weight of the muscles in the castrated male and increased muscle weights of the female. I confirmed a decrease in temporal muscle weight of the castrated male guinea pig and a growth-stimulating effect of testosterone propionate on the temporal muscle of the normal female and the castrated male guinea pig (Table 1.1) (Kochakian, Humm, & Bartlett, 1948). The increase in weight of the muscle was due to hypertrophy (Figure 1.4). The diameter of the cross section of the muscle fibers was much greater in the normal adult guinea pig than in the castrated guinea pig (Fig. 1.4). The diameter of the muscles of the treated guinea pigs was identical with that of the normal guinea pigs and is not shown. Furthermore, the total DNA, which is indicative of the number of cells, was not changed by castration or testosterone propionate treatment (Kochakian, Hill, & Harrison, 1964).

A comparison of the effectiveness of several steroids revealed that 5α-androstane-3α, 17β-diol produced a partial dichotomy between the growth of the muscle and the accessory sex organs. The study was then

**Table 1.1   Comparison of Temporal Muscle Weight (g)
of Adult Guinea Pigs and of the Effect of Testosterone Propionate**

Male			Female	
Normal	Castrated*	Castrated** plus TP	Normal	Normal** plus TP
2.08	0.98	1.80	0.54	1.01

*Castration was at approximately 400 g body weight. **Testosterone propionate (TP) was implanted subcutaneously as two 15 ± mg cylindrical pellets at the time of castration. The pellets were recovered at autopsy (54 days after castration), cleaned, dried, and weighed. The amount absorbed was 340 µg/day for the castrated males and 390 µg/day for the normal females.

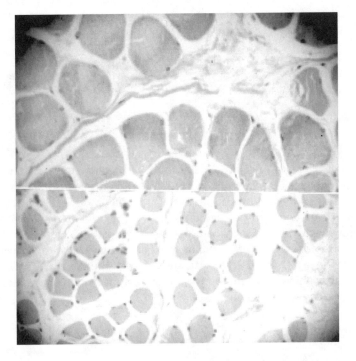

Figure 1.4   A comparison of the diameter of the fibers in the temporal muscle of the normal and castrated guinea pig. *Note.* Reprinted from Kochakian (1990a).

extended (Kochakian, 1975; Kochakian & Tillotson, 1957) to include 47 other muscles to determine the general nature of the response. The increase in size of the different muscles differed not only for the several steroids but also for the individual muscles. The sensitivity of the muscles to the steroids was greatest in the head and neck region and gradually diminished from head to hindquarters (Figure 1.5). Of further interest was the effect of 5α-dihydrotestosterone (5α-DHT). It was more active than testosterone in its androgenic effect and even more active in the myotrophic effect.

Rat: Skeletal Muscles

Castration of young rats (36 to 40 days of age) slightly decreased the rate of body growth and proportionately decreased the weight of practically all of the skeletal muscles (Kochakian, Tillotson, & Endahl, 1956). Our preliminary unpublished experiments with the injection of testosterone propionate and methyltestosterone did not produce any remarkable disproportionate increase in any of the many skeletal muscles but suggested a small increase in several of the muscles. Thompson, Boxhon, King, and Allen (1989) reported that the injection of trenbolone acetate (17β-acetoxy-3-oxo-estra-4,9,11-triene) at 80 µg per 100 g body weight per day for 14 days (initial body weight was 63 to 124 g) increased the rate of growth of female rats with no acceleration of the growth of the gastrocnemius, anterior tibialis, and peroneus complex muscles but a small increase in the growth of the semimembranosus muscle. The DNA of all of the muscles was increased.

Anabolic Steroids

Although a group of synthetically modified testosterone steroids have been popularized as anabolic steroids, there is no such thing as a pure anabolic steroid. All of the modified steroids still retain sufficient virilizing activity to make them objectionable as therapeutic agents especially in children and women. Furthermore, researchers have presumed but never demonstrated that the response of the levator ani (dorsal bulbocavernosus) muscle is representative of the responses of the skeletal muscles. This muscle is in fact one of the perineal complex muscles that are located in the pelvic cavity.

Levator Ani

Hershberger, Shipley, and Meyer (1953) used the suggestion of Eisenberg and Gordan (1950) to develop a quantitative assay procedure and found that 19-nortestosterone stimulated a greater response in the levator ani

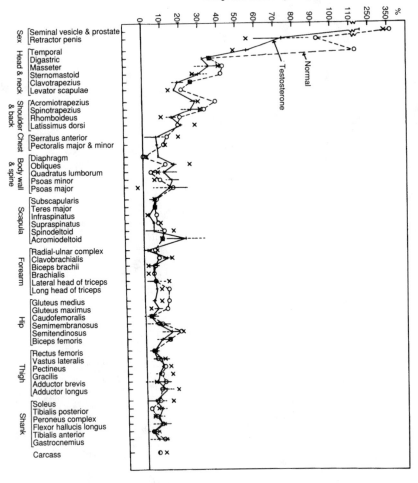

Figure 1.5 Response of the individual muscles of the castrated guinea pig to testosterone stimulation. Reprinted from Kochakian & Tillotson (1957) by permission.

muscle than in the accessory sex organs of the castrated rat. The authors presumed that the changes in weight of this muscle were representative of the skeletal muscles and designated its response to the steroids as anabolic, but this has not been proven (see sections on the muscles of guinea pigs and rats, pp. 14-16). The protein of the skeletal muscles of the rat represents approximately 60% of the protein of the body (Kochakian & Webster, 1958). The levator ani muscle proved to be the sex-linked dorsal bulbocavernosus muscle (Hayes, 1968; also see Nimni & Geiger, 1957), but the assay because of its simplicity, inexpensiveness, and use of the

Table 3.2 Self-Reported Anabolic Steroid Use Among Junior High and High School Students

Reference	Site and sample	N	Response rate (%)[a]	Incidence of use[a]		
				Grade	M	F	Total

Reference	Site and sample	N	Response rate (%)[a]	Grade	M	F	Total
Corder et al., 1975[b]	Arizona, 10 schools	1,393 (1971 survey)	—	—	—	—	0.7
		1,099 (1975 survey)	—	—	—	—	0.7
		208 athletes (1975 survey)	—	—	—	—	4
Newman, 1986[c]	Michigan, 11 school districts	5,029	—	8	—	—	3
				10	—	—	2
				12	5	1	2
Polen et al., 1986[b]	Florida, 1 school	200	—	9-12	18	0	—
Bosworth et al., 1987[b]	Oregon, 6 schools	190 athletes	—	9-12	1.1	—	—
Buckley et al., 1988[c]	24 states, 46 schools	3,403	50	12	6.6	—	—
Johnson et al., 1989[c]	Arkansas, 6 schools	1,775	99.5	11	11	0.5	5.7
Windsor & Dumitru, 1989[c]	Texas, 10 schools	901	89	9-12	5.0	1.4	3.0
Ross et al., 1989	Maryland, 215 schools	13,461	—	6	—	—	2.0
				8	—	—	2.3
				10	—	—	2.2
				12	4.6	1.4	3.1

(Cont.)

Table 3.2 (Continued)

Reference	Site and sample	N	Response rate (%)[a]	Incidence of use[a]			
				Grade	M	F	Total
Ringwalt, 1989	North Carolina	11,531	—	7	3.2	0.7	—
				8	3.1	0.5	—
				9	3.3	0.6	—
				10	3.3	0.5	—
				11	3.2	0.5	—
				12	3.0	0.3	—
Krowchuck et al., 1989	Ohio, 3 schools	295 athletes	99	9-12	—	—	1.4
Hubbel, 1990	Michigan, 12 schools	5,252	—	10	12	4	8
				12	12	4	8
Terney and McLain, 1990[b]	Illinois, 1 school	2,113	69	9	—	—	4.3
				10	—	—	4.8
				11	—	—	4.6
				12	—	—	4.2
				9-12	6.5	2.5	4.4
Vaughan et al., 1991	New York, 3 schools	119	92	9-10	15.3	6.7	10.9
Johnston et al., 1990	32 states, 133 schools	2,600	92	12	4.7	1.3	3.0
Johnston et al., 1991	34 states, 137 schools	2,350	86	12	5.0	.5	2.9
NIDA, 1991	50 states	874	84.2	12	—	—	2.5

[a]Dash indicates information was not reported.
[b]Reprinted from Yesalis, Anderson, Buckley, and Wright (1990).
[c]Reprinted from Yesalis, Wright, and Lombardo (1989) by permission.

Table 3.3 Self-Reported Anabolic Steroid Use Among College Students

Reference	Site and sample	N	Response rate (%)[a]	Incidence of use	
				Group	%
Dezelsky et al., 1985[b]	5 universities	4,171	—	Athletes, 1970	15
				Athletes, 1984	20
				Nonathletes, 1984	1
Anderson & McKeag, 1985[b]	11 universities, intercollegiate athletes	2,039	72	Football	9
				Division I	5
				Division II	4
				Division III	2
				Men's track and field	4
				Men's basketball	4
				Men's tennis	4
				Men's baseball	3
				Women's swimming	1

(Cont.)

Table 3.3 (Continued)

Reference	Site and sample	N	Response rate (%)[a]	Incidence of use Group	%
Anderson et al., 1991	11 universities, intercollegiate athletes	2,282	70	Football	10
				Division I	5
				Division II	5
				Division III	4
				Men's track and field	4
				Men's baseball	2
				Men's basketball	2
				Men's tennis	2
				Women's swimming	1
				Women's track and field	1
				Women's basketball	1
				Men overall	6.4
				Women overall	1
Pope et al., 1988[b]	3 universities	1,010	30	Men (Varsity athletes (n = 147)	2 9.4

[a]Dash indicates information was not reported.
[b]Reprinted from Yesalis, Wright, and Lombardo (1989) by permission.

Table 3.4 **Estimates of Anabolic Steroid Use During the Past 12 Months Among Division I National Collegiate Athletics Association Athletes (%) (Self-Reported vs. Projected Use)**

Reference			Male			
	Baseball	Basketball	Football	Tennis	Track and field	Weighted mean
Anderson et al., 1991	2.6	1.6	9.6	0	2.3	6.2
Yesalis, Buckley, et al., 1990	6.67	6.86	22.43	2.76	16.03	16.4

Reference			Female			
	Softball	Basketball	Swimming	Tennis	Track and field	Weighted mean
Anderson et al., 1991	0	0	0	0	1.5	0.6
Yesalis, Buckley, et al., 1990	2.92	6.25	5.35	5.60	9.53	6.37

All sports, male and female combined

Reference	
Anderson et al., 1991 (Self-reported use)	4.8
Yesalis, Buckley, et al., 1990 (Projected use)	14.06

Note. From Yesalis, Buckley, et al. (1990). Used by permission.

Table 3.5 Self-Reported Anabolic Steroid Use Among Other Athletes

Reference	Site and sample	N [a]	Response rate (%) [a]	Incidence of use Group	Incidence of use %
Silvester, 1973	1972 Olympians in track and field from 7 countries	—	—	Total	68
				Past 6 months	61
Ljungqvist, 1975[b]	Elite Swedish male track-and-field athletes	99	69	Total	31
				Throwers	75
				Middle- and long-distance runners	0
Newman, 1987[b]	Elite female athletes in over 15 sports	271	59	Total	3
				Past 12 months	1
Yesalis et al., 1988[b]	Elite power lifters	45	74	Questionnaire ($n = 45$)	33
				Follow-up phone contact ($n = 20$)	55
Frankle et al., 1984[b]	Weight trainers in 3 gymnasiums	250	—	Total	44
McKillop, 1987	Male amateur bodybuilders in 1 gymnasium	41	—	Total	19.5
Tricker et al., 1989	Amateur competitive bodybuilders in Missouri and Kansas	176	46	M ($n = 108$)	54.6
				F ($n = 68$)	10
Kisling et al., 1989	Bodybuilders in 1 gymnasium	138	—	M	62
Lindstrum et al., 1990	Swedish bodybuilders in 1 gymnasium	171	90	M ($n = 138$)	38.4
				F ($n = 33$)	9.1
Yesalis & Courson, 1990	NFL players	120	7.5	Lifetime	28
				Past 12 months	3

[a]Dash indicates information was not reported.

[b]Reprinted from Yesalis, Wright, and Lombardo (1989) by permission.

In 1987 the first nationwide study of anabolic steroid use at the high school level was conducted by Buckley, Yesalis, Friedl, Anderson, Streit, & Wright (1988), who found that 6.6% of male high school seniors reported having used these drugs (Table 3.2). There was no difference in the levels of reported anabolic steroid use between urban and rural areas, but there was a small but significant difference by size of enrollment: Students at larger high schools had a higher rate of reported anabolic steroid use. Almost 40% of the anabolic steroid users reported five or more cycles of use. In addition, of the self-reported anabolic steroid users, 38% had initiated use before age 16, 44% used more than one steroid at a time (stacking), and 38% used injectable anabolic steroids. More than one-third of the anabolic steroid users did not intend to participate in interscholastic sports. Only 15% of the public and private high schools that participated in this study had no reported anabolic steroid use. However, in a survey of 472 head football coaches in Michigan high schools, only 12% admitted that they knew of at least one player who used anabolic steroids before 1988—or suspected as much (Duda, 1988).

Seven state-level studies confirm the findings of Buckley et al. (1988) and generally show that 5% to 12% of high school males admit having used anabolic steroids at some time (Hubbell, 1990; Johnson, Jay, Shoup, & Rickert, 1989; Ringwalt, 1989; Ross, Winters, Hartmann, Robb, & Dillemuth, 1989; Terney & McLain, 1990; Windsor & Dumitru, 1989; Vaughan, Walter, & Gladis, 1991). These seven studies also examined use of anabolic steroids among high school females and found that approximately 1 to 2% reported using steroids (Table 3.2). By contrast, one study of 295 high school athletes, including males, reported only a 1.4% prevalence of steroid use, although distributing the questionnaire during a preparticipation examination may have led to underreporting (Krowchuk et al., 1989). Recently two additional national surveys of high school seniors showed that approximately 3% (5.0% of males and 0.5 to 1% of females) acknowledged previous use of anabolic steroids; use in the prior 30 days was 1.4 to 1.7% and 0.1 to 0.3% in males and females, respectively (Johnston, Bachman, & O'Malley, 1990, 1991). The results of the 1991 National Household Survey on Drug Abuse (National Institute on Drug Abuse, 1991) showed the percent of high school seniors who had ever used steroids was only slightly less than that reported in the surveys described previously, with a prior use rate of 2.5% (sex-specific use rates were not available at the time of this writing).

College

Of 67 intercollegiate swimmers (male and female) from six universities surveyed in 1981, only one athlete (a male) reported prior use of anabolic steroids (Toohey & Corder, 1981). Dezelsky, Toohey, and Shaw (1985), in a study of nonmedical drug use among students at five public universities in 1970 and 1984, found that only 1% of nonathlete students reported using anabolic steroids in 1984. However, the percentage of intercollegiate athletes who reported anabolic steroid use rose from 15% in 1970 to 20% in 1984 (Table 3.3). Anabolic steroid use rates were not reported separately for males and females, nor were they reported by sport.

Anderson and McKeag (1985) surveyed 2,039 NCAA male and female athletes at 11 NCAA member colleges and universities nationwide regarding alcohol and drug use (Table 3.3). The heaviest anabolic steroid use (defined as use in the past 12 months) was among football players (9%), whereas 4% of the male track-and-field athletes reported prior use. Men's sports not typically associated with anabolic steroid use but found to have some anabolic steroid users were baseball (3%), basketball (4%), and tennis (4%). For women, only one sport was associated with anabolic steroid use—swimming (1%). Overall, 5% of Division I athletes, 4% of Division II athletes, and 2% of Division III athletes reported anabolic steroid use in the year prior to the survey.

Anderson, Albrecht, McKeag, Hough, and McGrew (1991) replicated the Anderson and McKeag (1985) study of athletes during the 1988-89 academic year (Table 3.3). Data were collected from 2,282 male and female athletes at 11 colleges and universities. Seven of the original eleven universities participated in the second study. Overall, anabolic steroid use had increased only slightly over the preceding 4 years. For Division I athletes, reported anabolic steroid use remained at 5%. However, for Division II and Division III athletes, anabolic steroid use rose to 5% and 4%, respectively.

Across Divisions I-III, the highest incidence of reported anabolic steroid use was again among football players (10%). Anabolic steroid use remained the same for men's track and field (4%), but declined in baseball (2%), basketball (2%), and tennis (2%). Unlike the Anderson and McKeag (1985) study, which found anabolic steroid use in only one sport for women, the Anderson et al. (1991) survey revealed three women's sports associated with anabolic steroid use: track and field (1%), basketball (1%), and swimming (1%). Refer to Table 3.4 for Division I use rates for selected sports. For those athletes using steroids, 25% began use before college, 25% initiated use during the 1st year of college, and 50% began after the 1st year of college (Anderson et al., 1991).

Of the 1,010 respondents in a survey of college men at three eastern universities, 2% acknowledged anabolic steroid use, whereas 9.4% of the 147 varsity athletes in the sample reported using these drugs (Pope, Katz, & Champoux, 1988; Table 3.3).

Yesalis, Buckley, et al. (1990) employed projected-response survey techniques with collegiate athletes and used indirect questions. Thus respondents were asked to estimate the level of their competitors' steroid use. Over 1,600 male and female athletes at five NCAA Division I institutions participated in this study during the 1989-90 academic year. The mean overall projected rate of any prior use of anabolic steroids across all sports surveyed was 14.7% for male athletes and 5.9% for females. Among men's sports, football reported the highest projected lifetime anabolic steroid use rates with 29.3%, followed by track and field with 20.6%. The greatest projected steroid use rate for women's sports was for track and field (16.3%). The overall projected rate of steroid use during the past 12 months reported was approximately 3 times greater than the rate obtained from self-reports by Anderson and colleagues (1991) (Table 3.4).

Other Athletes

Silvester (1973) surveyed track-and-field athletes who participated in the 1972 Olympics and found that 68% of the participants reported prior anabolic steroid use, with 61% having used steroids within 6 months of the games (Table 3.5). In 1975 Ljungqvist surveyed elite Swedish male track-and-field athletes and found that 31% admitted prior anabolic steroid use (Ljungqvist, 1975). None of the middle- or long-distance runners admitted anabolic steroid use, but 75% of the throwers did (Table 3.5). In a survey of 155 U.S. Olympians who participated in the 1992 Winter Games, 80% of the athletes classified steroid use among Olympic competitors as a very serious or somewhat serious problem; just 5% thought that it was not a problem (Pearson & Hansen, 1992). When asked to estimate the level of steroid use in their own sport, 43% of the respondents estimated 10% or more, while 34% estimated 1 to 9%. Only 23% of the athletes surveyed believed that there was no steroid use in their sport.

Newman (1987) surveyed elite female athletes in more than 15 sports and found that lifetime incidence of anabolic steroid use was 3%, but only 1% of the athletes acknowledged using these drugs in the preceding year (Table 3.5). The lifetime use rate was slightly higher for those over the age of 26 (4%) and members of professional teams (5%).

In 1988, Yesalis et al. surveyed elite power lifters at a major contest, using both questionnaires and follow-up telephone interviews. One-third of the questionnaire respondents admitted prior anabolic steroid use, but 55% of those interviewed later by telephone conceded steroid use (Table 3.5).

Frankle, Cicero, and Payne (1984) questioned weight trainers in three gymnasiums in the Chicago area and found that 44% reported prior anabolic steroid use (Table 3.5). Of a subsample of 50 anabolic steroid users interviewed in-depth, only 44% were competing in athletics. Anabolic steroid use rates by sex were not reported. In 1985 McKillop surveyed bodybuilders in a gymnasium in Scotland, and 19.5% acknowledged prior steroid use (McKillop, 1987; Table 3.5). In a study of amateur competitive bodybuilders, over half of the men and 10% of the women reported using anabolic steroids at some time in their lives (Tricker, O'Neill, & Cook, 1989; Table 3.5). Similarly, two single-gym studies of bodybuilders revealed high lifetime use rates among men (62% and 38.4%) (Kisling, Fauner, Larsen, & Nielsen, 1989; Lindstrom, Nilsson, Katzman, Janzon, & Dymling, 1990; Table 3.5). A relatively high rate of anabolic steroid use (9.1%) was reported by female bodybuilders in one of these studies (Lindstrom et al., 1990). Among women, then, bodybuilders appear to have the highest self-reported rates of steroid use.

In 1990, an attempt was made to survey 1,600 NFL players via mail by the NFL Players Association and the Olympia Steele Management Group (Yesalis & Courson, 1990; Table 3.5). Only 120 players ($\approx$ 7.5%) elected to participate, however. Twenty-eight percent of all respondents and 67% of offensive linemen reported prior use of anabolic steroids. Only 3% of the participants reported steroid use in the past 12 months. When the participants were asked what percent of their fellow NFL players did they believe had ever used anabolic steroids, the mean response was 32%; the estimate of use among fellow players for the past 12 months was 19%.

Methodological Issues

The extent to which the respondents in these surveys honestly reported their anabolic steroid use is not known. It is possible that they intentionally underreported or overreported their anabolic steroid use. Intentional over-reporters could be characterized as braggarts who overemphasize drug use to present themselves in a more worldly manner. This is unlikely to be a major source of bias, however, because virtually all surveys dealing with anabolic steroid use are written and anonymous. Reasons for unintentional reporting errors include faulty memory, reading levels of the respondents, inability to understand the reporting time frames for drug use, and the complexity of the scales for reporting frequencies and amounts of drug use.

The research on the use of self-report methods has shown them to be valid for documenting recreational drug use, especially for adolescents (McClary & Lubin, 1985; Smart & Blair, 1978). When the recreational drug use rates from self-report studies have been compared with external methods of documenting drug use (e.g., reports by others, or blood and urine samples), the self-report use rates have been similar to or only slightly lower than the rates derived by the other methods (Ausel et al., 1976; Bonito, Nucro, & Schaffer, 1976; Deaux & Callaghen, 1984; Petzel, Johnson, & McKillip, 1973; Stacy, Widaman, & Hays, 1985). However, accuracy of reporting as it is applied to adolescent steroid use is brought into question by the results of a study of high school athletes in 1988 (Krowchuk et al., 1989). Among the participants 39% of male athletes and

56% of females denied that they had even heard of anabolic steroid use as a performance aid; this study took place during a decade that was marked by significant media attention to drug use among athletes (Wadler & Hainline, 1989). Moreover, in the survey of elite (adult) power lifters described previously, only 33% reported having ever used anabolic steroids (Yesalis et al., 1988), this in a sport in which many believe the use of these drugs is virtually universal (Starr, 1981; Todd, 1987; Wright, 1982). When a co-investigator whom the study participants knew again questioned (via telephone) some of the lifters on their steroid use, 55% admitted prior use. Thus it is possible that the level of trust the subjects felt with the interviewer was a more important factor to them than anonymity.

The apparent discrepancy between adolescents' willingness to report drug use and the hesitancy of the power lifters (and perhaps other adult athletes) might be explained in several ways. Adolescents possibly have less to lose than college, elite, or professional athletes whose scholarships or livelihoods depend on their participation and success in sport. Thus, the respondents in the studies of athletes reviewed here may have under-reported their drug use to meet more socially acceptable standards of behavior (Dillman, 1978). The use of anabolic steroids violates not only the rules of virtually all sport federations but also the traditional ethics of fair play in sports; steroid use would likely meet with the disapproval of family, friends, and fans. Indeed, even though these surveys guaranteed personal anonymity, the subjects might have underreported because of concern for the reputations of their schools or athletic conferences. Another problem that is perhaps inherent in anonymous studies of drug use in athletics is that these studies can harm the reputation of the sport. The fear of guilt by association and its potential to adversely affect the athlete's place in sport history may result in a hesitancy to volunteer or be truthful. The difficulty of convincing athletes to be open about steroid use has been depicted as "getting only a glimpse of a large underground subculture" (Pope & Katz, 1988, p. 489). Furthermore, the *Commission of Inquiry Into the Use of Drugs and Banned Practices Intended to Increase Athletic Performance* (Dubin, 1990) uses the term "conspiracy of silence" when describing the hesitation or refusal of athletes and sport officials to discuss steroid use. Because of the virilizing qualities of anabolic steroids (Kochakian, 1976), women might be more secretive about their anabolic steroid use than men or adolescents.

Any underreporting of anabolic steroid use among postadolescent athletes might also be due, in part, to the lack of trust and communication between members of the athletic community and the scientific and medical communities. This, in turn, is a function of poor understanding on the part of researchers and physicians of the motivations of athletes, and vice versa (Duchaine, 1989). The medical community has lost much credibility as a result of repeated denials that steroids enhance performance (ACSM, 1977; Council on Scientific Affairs, AMA, 1990). Until recently, physicians and scientists dogmatically reported that any weight that an athlete gained while taking steroids was mainly the result of fluid retention and that any strength gain was largely psychological (a placebo effect). This credibility gap has been exacerbated by the apparent contradiction between the medical community's warnings of resultant dire health consequences of steroid use by athletes and the current 10-center worldwide trial sponsored by the World Health Organization to test the efficacy of anabolic steroids in male contraception (World Health Organization Task Force on Methods for the Regulation of Male Fertility, 1990; "Male Contraceptive Use," 1990).

The response rates of the studies reviewed here ranged from 7.5 to 99.5% or were not reported. We have no information on individuals who chose not to volunteer information, but we can hypothesize that a disproportionate number of those who did not participate were anabolic steroid users, which would result in an underreporting bias.

It is reasonable to infer that the level of anabolic steroid use as determined by the self-report survey method likely reflects a lower bound and that the level of underreporting may vary by age, sport, level of competition, and sex.

On the other hand, indirect survey techniques (i.e., in which respondents estimate their competitors' anabolic steroid use level) rely to some extent on hearsay as well as the opportunity to project one's own behavior on others, and the resulting estimates of use probably represent an upper bound or overestimation of use (Tricker et al., 1989; Yesalis, Buckley, et al., 1990). This indirect survey method is probably less threatening to the athlete in that it does not require the respondent to divulge information about himself or herself or about specific teammates; this method likely results in a higher level of participation in the study. Undoubtedly a certain amount of projection also takes place (Semeonoff, 1976). That is, the respondent protects himself or herself from anxiety by projecting or externalizing inappropriate behaviors to others, as if by projecting these behaviors (in this case anabolic steroid use) to someone else, one denies or rationalizes their existence within oneself. Also, anxiety related to one's own inappropriate behavior may be diluted if the behavior can be projected toward others in an effort to characterize the activity as less atypical or more mainstream. Thus the true level of anabolic steroid use among athletes probably lies between the lower-bound estimates from self-reports and the upper-bound estimates obtained from the projective response techniques.

Another issue that deserves comment is the number of studies that give attention in their analyses to any prior steroid use rather than focusing solely on use within the past 12 months. Anabolic steroids are not necessarily temporary performance enhancers; they are capable of providing the athlete with increased muscle mass and strength, some of which can be maintained for a number of years through training alone. One might then argue that once you use anabolic steroids you are never really the same person. Consequently, is there a difference between a college football player who does not currently use steroids but used them in high school to gain enough weight to obtain a scholarship and a college player who used the drugs during the past season to maintain his starting position?

Conclusion

The level of anabolic steroid use has increased significantly over the past 3 decades, and it is no longer limited to elite athletes or men. Although higher rates of anabolic steroid use are reported by competitive athletes, a significant number of recreational athletes appear to be using these drugs, probably to improve their appearance. The use of anabolic steroids has trickled down from the Olympic, professional, and college levels to the high schools and the junior high schools. Steroid use has been reported by adolescents in both urban and rural areas and in schools of all sizes, and it is believed that among high school seniors, between 5 and 12% of males and 0.5 to 2% of females have used anabolic steroids at some time.

The results of drug tests at athletic events are a poor indicator of the overall incidence of anabolic steroid use. Likewise, the results of surveys based on self-reports likely represent a lower-bound of the level of steroid use.

References

American College of Sports Medicine. (1977). Position statement on the use and abuse of anabolic-androgenic steroids in sports. *Medicine and Science in Sports and Exercise,* **9,** 11-13.

Anderson, W.A., Albrecht, M.A., McKeag, D.B., Hough, D.O., & McGrew, C.A. (1991). A national survey of alcohol and drug use by college athletes. *The Physician and Sportsmedicine,* **19**(2), 91-104.

Anderson, W., & McKeag, D. (1985). *The substance use and abuse habits of college student-athletes* (Research Paper No. 2). Mission, KS: National Collegiate Athletic Association.

Ausel, S., Mandell, W., Mathias, L., et al. (1976). Reliability and validity of self-reported illegal activities and drug use collected from narcotic addicts. *International Journal of the Addictions,* **11,** 325-336.

Bonito, A., Nucro, D., & Schaffer, J. (1976). The verdicality of addicts' self-reports in social research. *International Journal of the Addictions,* **11,** 719-724.

Bosworth, E., Bents, R., Trevisan, L., & Goldberg, L. (1987). Anabolic steroids and high school athletes. *Medicine and Science in Sports and Exercise*, **20**(2) (Suppl.), S3, 17.

Buckley, W., Yesalis, C., Friedl, K., Anderson, W., Streit, A., & Wright, J. (1988). Estimated prevalence of anabolic steroid use among male high school seniors. *Journal of the American Medical Association*, **260**, 3441-3445.

Catlin, D. (1987). Detection of drug use by athletes. In R.H. Strauss (Ed.), *Drugs and performance in sports* (pp. 103-120). Philadelphia: Saunders.

Catlin, D., Kammerer, R., Hatton, C., et al. (1987). Analytical chemistry at the games of the XXIIIrd Olympiad in Los Angeles. *Clinical Chemistry*, **33**, 319-327.

Catlin, D.H., & Hatton, C.K. (1991). Use and abuse of anabolic and other drugs for athletic enhancement. *Advances in Internal Medicine*, **36**, 399-424.

Corder, B.W., Dezelsky, T.L., Toohey, J.V., & DiVito, C.L. (1975). Trends in drug use behavior at ten Central Arizona high schools. *Arizona Journal of Health, Physical Education, Recreation and Dance*, **18**, 10-11.

Council on Scientific Affairs, American Medical Association. (1990). Medical and nonmedical uses of anabolic-androgenic steroids. *Journal of the American Medical Association*, **264**, 2923-2927.

Cowart, V. (1988). Accord on drug testing, sanctions sought before 1992 Olympics in Europe. *Journal of the American Medical Association*, **260**, 3397-3398.

deMerode, A. (1988, April). Unpublished letter, International Medical Commission Code of Ethics for IOC Accredited Laboratories. Lucerne, Switzerland, International Medical Commission.

Deaux, E., & Callaghen, J. (1984). Estimating statewide health risk behavior: A comparison of telephone and key information survey approaches. *Evaluation Review*, **8**, 467-492.

Dezelsky, T., Toohey, J., & Shaw, R. (1985). Non-medical drug use behavior at five United States universities: A 15-year study. *Bulletin on Narcotics*, **27**, 45-53.

Dillman, D. (1978). *Mail and telephone surveys*. New York: Wiley.

Di Pasquale, M.G. (1984). *Drug use and detection in amateur sports*. Warkworth, ON: M.G.D. Press.

Dubin, C. (1990). *Commission of inquiry into the use of drugs and banned practices intended to increase athletic performance* (Catalogue No. CP32-56/1990E, ISBN 0-660-13610-4). Ottawa, ON: Canadian Government Publishing Center.

Duchaine, D. (1989). *Underground steroid handbook II*. Venice, CA: HLR Technical Books.

Duda, M. (1988). Gauging steroid use in high school kids. *The Physician and Sportsmedicine*, **16**, 16-17.

Francis, C. (1990). *Speed trap*. New York: St. Martin's Press.

Frankle, M., Cicero, G., & Payne, J. (1984). Use of androgenic anabolic steroids by athletes [Letter to the editor]. *Journal of the American Medical Association, 252*, 482.

Frazier, S. (1973). Androgens and athletes. *American Journal of Diseases of Children, 125*, 479-480.

Friedl, K., Jones, R., Hannan, C., & Plymate, S. (1989). The administration of pharmacological doses of testosterone or 19-nortestosterone to normal men is not associated with increased insulin secretion or impaired glucose tolerance. *Journal of Clinical Endocrinology and Metabolism, 68*, 971-975.

Gilbert, B. (1969a, June 23). Drugs in sport: Part 1. Problems in a turned-on world. *Sports Illustrated*, pp. 64-72.

Gilbert, B. (1969b, June 30). Drugs in sport: Part 2. Something extra on the ball. *Sports Illustrated*, pp. 30-42.

Gilbert, B. (1969c, July 7). Drugs in sport: Part 3. High time to make some rules. *Sports Illustrated*, pp. 30-35.

Goldman, B. (1984). *Death in the locker room*. South Bend, IN: Icarus Press.

Hubbell, N. (1990). *The use of steroids by Michigan high school students and athletes: An opinion research study of 10th and 12th grade high school students and varsity athletes, November 1989 through January 1990*. Lansing: Michigan Department of Public Health, Chronic Disease Advisory Committee.

Janofsky, M. (1988, November 17). System accused of failing test posed by drugs. *New York Times*.

Johnson, M., Jay, M., Shoup, B., & Rickert, V. (1989). Anabolic steroid use in adolescent males. *Pediatrics, 83*, 921-924.

Johnston, L., Bachman, J., O'Malley, P. (1990). *Monitoring the future: Continuing study of the lifestyles and values of youth*. Ann Arbor: University of Michigan Institute for Social Research.

Johnston, L., Bachman, J., & O'Malley, P. (1991). *Monitoring the future: Continuing study of the lifestyles and values of youth*. Ann Arbor: University of Michigan Institute for Social Research.

Kisling, A., Fauner, M., Larsen, O.G., & Nielsen, S. (1989). Medicinmisbrug blandt bodybuildere. *Journal of Danish Medicine, 151*, 2582-2584.

Kochakian, C. (Ed.) (1976). *Anabolic-androgenic steroids*. New York: Springer-Verlag.

Krowchuk, D., Anglin, T., Goodfellow, D., Stancin, T., Williams, P., & Zimet, G. (1989). High school athletes and the use of ergogenic aids. *American Journal of Diseases of Children, 143*, 486-489.

Lindstrom, M., Nilsson, A., Katzman, P., Janzon, L., & Dymling, J. (1990). Use of anabolic-androgenic steroids among body builders—frequency and attitudes. *Journal of Internal Medicine, 227*, 407-411.

Ljungqvist, A. (1975). The use of anabolic steroids in top Swedish athletes. *British Journal of Sports Medicine, 9*, 82.

Male contraceptive use: Safe and effective steroid use. (1990, November-December). *Anabolic Reference Update, 22.* [Available from Mile High Publishing, Golden, CO].

McClary, S., & Lubin, B. (1985). Effects of type of examiner, sex, and year in school on self-report of drug use by high school students. *Journal of Drug Education, 15,* 49-55.

McKillop, G. (1987). Drug abuse in bodybuilders in the west of Scotland. *Scottish Medical Journal, 32,* 39-41.

National Institute on Drug Abuse. (1991). *National Household survey on drug abuse: Population estimates, 1991.* Rockville, MD: U.S. Department of Health and Human Services; Public Health Service; Alcohol, Drug Abuse, and Mental Health Administration. DHHS Publication No. ADM-92-1887.

Newman, M. (1986). *Michigan Consortium of Schools student survey.* Minneapolis, MN: Hazelden Research Services.

Newman, M. (1987). *Elite women athletes survey results.* Center City, MN: Hazelden Research Services.

Pearson, B., & Hansen, B. (1992, February 5). Survey of U.S. Olympians. *USA Today,* p. 10C.

Petzel, T., Johnson, J., & McKillip, J. (1973). Response bias in drug surveys. *Journal of Consulting and Clinical Psychology, 40,* 437-439.

Polen, L., Shnider, L., Sirotowitz, A., & West, J. (1986, October). Teenage drug epidemics: Build up on steroids. *Sword and Shield.* [Available from South Plantation High School, Broward County, FL]

Pope, H., & Katz, D. (1988). Affective and psychotic symptoms associated with anabolic steroid use. *American Journal of Psychiatry, 145,* 487-490.

Pope, H., Katz, D., & Champoux, R. (1988). Anabolic-androgenic steroid use among 1,010 college men. *The Physician and Sportsmedicine, 16,* 75-81.

Ringwalt, C. (1989). *Alcohol and other drug use patterns among students in North Carolina public schools, grades 7-12: Results of a 1989 student survey.* Raleigh: North Carolina Department of Public Instruction, Alcohol and Drug Defense Section, Division of Student Services.

Ross, J., Winters, F., Hartmann, K., Robb, W., & Dillemuth, K. (1989). *1988-89 survey of substance abuse among Maryland adolescents.* Baltimore: Maryland Department of Health and Mental Hygiene, Alcohol and Drug Abuse Administration.

Semeonoff, B. (1976). *Projective techniques.* London: Wiley.

Silvester, L. (1973). Anabolic steroids at the 1972 Olympics. *Scholastic Coach, 43,* 90-92.

Smart, R., & Blair, N. (1978). Test-retest reliability and validity information for a high school drug use questionnaire. *Drug and Alcohol Dependence, 3,* 265-271.

Stacy, A., Widaman, K., & Hays, R. (1985). Validity of self-reports of alcohol and other drug use. A multitrait-multimethod assessment. *Journal of Personality and Social Psychology, 49,* 219-232.

Starr, B. (1981). *Defying gravity: How to win at weightlifting.* Wichita Falls, TX: Five Starr Productions.

Terney, R., & McLain, L. (1990). The use of anabolic steroids in high school students. *American Journal of Diseases of Children, 144,* 99-103.

Todd, T. (1987). Anabolic steroids: The gremlins of sport. *Journal of Sport History, 14,* 87-107.

Toohey, J., & Corder, B. (1981). Intercollegiate sports participation and nonmedical drug use. *Bulletin on Narcotics, 23*(3), 23-26.

Tricker, R., O'Neill, M., & Cook, D. (1989). The incidence of anabolic steroid use among competitive bodybuilders. *Journal of Drug Education, 19*(4), 313-325.

Vaughan, R., Walter, H., & Gladis, M. (1991). Steroid use among adolescents—Another look. *AIDS, 5,* 112-113.

Voy, R. (1990). *Drugs, sport, and politics.* Champaign, IL: Leisure Press.

Wade, N. (1972). Anabolic steroids: Doctors denounce them, but athletes aren't listening. *Science, 176,* 1399-1403.

Wadler, G., & Hainline, B. (1989). *Drugs and the athlete.* Philadelphia: Davis.

Windsor, R., & Dumitru, D. (1989). Anabolic steroid use by adolescents: Survey. *Medicine and Science in Sports and Exercise, 21,* 494-497.

World Health Organization Task Force on Methods for the Regulation of Male Fertility. (1990). Contraceptive efficacy of testosterone-induced azoospermia in normal men. *Lancet, 336,* 955-959.

Wright, J. (1978). *Anabolic steroids and sports.* Natick, MA: Sports Science Consultants.

Wright, J. (1982). *Anabolic steroids and sports II.* Natick, MA: Sports Science Consultants.

Yesalis, C.E., Anderson, W.A., Buckley, W.E., & Wright, J.E. (1990). Incidence of the nonmedical use of anabolic-androgenic steroids. In G. Lin & L. Erinoff (Eds.), *Anabolic steroid abuse* (National Institute on Drug Abuse Research, Monograph 102, DHHS Publication No. ADM 90-1720). Rockville, MD: U.S. Department of Health and Human Services, Public Health Service.

Yesalis, C.E., Buckley, W.A., Anderson, W.A., Wang, M.O., Norwig, J.A., Ott, G., Puffer, J.C., & Strauss, R.H. (1990). Athletes' projections of anabolic steroid use. *Clinical Sports Medicine, 2,* 155-171.

Yesalis, C.E., & Courson, S.P. (1990). [Anabolic steroid use among a self-selected sample of NFL players], Unpublished data.

Yesalis, C., Herrick, R., Buckley, W., Friedl, K., Brannon, D., & Wright, J. (1988). Self-reported use of anabolic-androgenic steroids by elite power lifters. *The Physician and Sportsmedicine, 16,* 91-100.

Yesalis, C.E., Wright, J.E., & Lombardo, J.A. (1989). Anabolic-androgenic steroids: A synthesis of existing data and recommendations for future research. *Clinical Sports Medicine, 1,* 109-134.

CHAPTER 4

A Study of Anabolic Steroid Use at the Secondary School Level: Recommendations for Prevention

W.E. Buckley
Charles E. Yesalis
David L. Bennell

I think they are virtually worthless, but everybody uses them [steroids] before contests—so I do too.

ARNOLD SCHWARZENEGGER
Sports Illustrated, October 14, 1974, p. 120

Portions of this chapter are reprinted from Streit and Wright (1988) by permission; see credits page for more information.

The 1988 study described in this chapter represents the first nationwide survey of anabolic steroid use among the general adolescent male population. Impetus for the development of this study was provided by several of the early regional studies mentioned in chapter 3 and by anecdotal accounts from high school athletes, coaches, and athletic administrators that suggested that anabolic steroid use was much more widespread than previously documented.

Methods

Study Population

Participants in this investigation were 12th-grade male students in private and public high schools. We selected this population because of a priori evidence that this group made up a significant portion of users within the general adolescent population. According to Jessor's concept of developmental transition, problem behaviors such as illicit drug abuse play a key role in the lives and behavior patterns of this age group (English, 1987; Jessor, 1982). It has been postulated that a significant proportion of the developmental transition has occurred by the time a student reaches the 12th grade, and we believe that students in this grade make up the best study population.

We drew a sample of schools from a pool of 150 high schools across the nation that employed certified athletic trainers who had participated in a sports epidemiology survey within the prior 2 years (Powell, 1987). (A certified athletic trainer is a professional who has graduated from an accredited institution and has successfully completed a certification examination administered by a testing agency for the National Athletic Trainers Association, Inc. This association is a member of the National Commission for Health Certifying Agencies. Certified athletic trainers are generally based in high schools, universities, and professional athletics, and their primary responsibilities are prevention, recognition, treatment, and rehabilitation of athletic injuries.)

The 150 schools in this study do not represent a random sample of all high schools in the United States, because only 12% of high schools employ certified athletic trainers. Our sample schools, however, do share the characteristics of a large number of schools in this country. We stratified these high schools into eight categories (or cells; Table 4.1) based on general demographic characteristics:

- urban (metropolitan statistical area) versus rural (nonmetropolitan statistical area) locales,
- large (>700 students) versus small (<700 students) enrollments, and
- Sunbelt versus non-Sunbelt locales.

Sunbelt locale was defined as contiguous states that border any ocean body or Mexico from Virginia south and west to Texas, Arizona, New Mexico, and California. The strata were selected based on anecdotal accounts that the rate of steroid use is higher among students in large, urban schools in Sunbelt states.

We drew a random proportional sample of schools within each of the eight categories. The schools were treated as clusters of potential respondents, and all male seniors were invited to participate. All Sunbelt schools with enrollments less than 700 and rural Sunbelt schools with enrollments more than 700 were used due to the small numbers available in these pools.

The athletic trainer at each school was contacted by the principal investigators and asked to collaborate on the study. In total, 46 of the 67 schools contacted completed the study protocol, for a return rate of 68.7%. Out of 6,765 male senior students who were eligible from the responding institutions, 3,403 (50.3%) voluntarily participated.

Data Collection

A questionnaire was employed to collect the data. All the respondents completed the first section of the instrument, which consisted of 11 questions, the last of which established current or previous use of anabolic steroids. Those who answered *yes* to this question were instructed to proceed to a series of 12 questions that further explored steroid usage. Those who responded *no* were directed to 12 questions related to basic health behavior. This strategy likely resulted in equal survey completion times for steroid users and nonusers, helping to assure anonymity during the administration of the instrument. Pilot surveys established that the instrument could be used with this population without difficulty and required similar amounts of time for both users and nonusers of steroids to complete.

The questionnaires were administered to all male seniors by their homeroom teachers. This setting provided a normal testing environment and was used for completion of all the surveys. The investigators maintained confidentiality by having the homeroom teachers seal the collection envelopes before returning them to the athletic trainer, who then forwarded them to the researchers for scoring and tabulation.

The tabular analysis involved simple frequency counts and percentages. The X^2 statistic was used to test for significant differences between groups, primarily between anabolic steroid users and nonusers.

Table 4.1 Stratification

Characteristic	Cell							
	1	2	3	4	5	6	7	8
Sunbelt?	Yes	No	Yes	No	Yes	No	Yes	No
Statistical area	Metro	Metro	Metro	Metro	Non-metro	Non-metro	Non-metro	Non-metro
Total no. of students in each school	>700	>700	<700	<700	>700	>700	<700	<700
No. of schools contacted	9	14	5	10	6	10	3	10
No. and percent of schools that participated	2 (22.2)	10 (71.4)	3 (60.0)	8 (80.0)	4 (66.7)	8 (80.0)	1 (33.3)	10 (100.0)
Total male enrollment in participating schools	450	2466	398	614	703	1196	20	918
No. and percent of questionnaires returned	224 (49.8)	1152 (46.7)	174 (43.7)	342 (55.7)	352 (50.1)	656 (54.8)	20 (100)	446 (48.6)

Note. Metro = metropolitan; Non-metro = non-metropolitan. Forms for 32 respondents could not be linked to an institution. These subjects are not included in this table but are included in all analyses. Reprinted from Buckley et al. (1988) by permission.

Results

The mean rate of anabolic steroid use for the entire sample, with the school as the unit of analysis, was 6.34% ± 5.61% ($N = 46$); with the student as the unit of analysis a mean use rate of 6.64% (226/3403) was derived. In interpreting the data we considered both of these rates to account for possible "nesting" effects related to the stratification (Whiting-O'Keefe, Henke, & Simborg, 1984). These data indicate that the nesting effects were negligible (calculation of a weighted mean of 6.41% demonstrates a small nesting effect of school size) and not at all confounding, because in either case, between 6 and 7 individuals out of 100 reported current or previous use of anabolic steroids. However, the results indicate significant variation among the participating institutions, with seven schools (15%) reporting no steroid use.

The test for dependence between steroid use and sampling strata (metropolitan statistical area designation, enrollment, and locale) showed only enrollment to be associated with use/nonuse behavior ($p<.05$). Although schools with greater than 700 students made up 69.6% of the sample, 76.1% of the users attended the larger schools.

Although all respondents were males in the 12th grade, subjects in the user group tended to be chronologically older (>19 years) ($p<.001$) (Table 4.2). The racial composition also differed between user and nonuser groups, with greater minority representation in the user group ($p<.001$). In addition, respondents in the nonuser group were more likely to have a parent who finished high school ($p<.001$).

Participation in sports activities was significantly different between users and nonusers, with the users more inclined to participate in school-sponsored athletics ($p<.05$) and, specifically, more likely to participate in football and wrestling (Table 4.3). More revealing was that 35.2% of the user group did not intend to participate in a school-sponsored activity.

Two questions were specifically designed to differentiate between the attitudes and self-perceptions of the users and nonusers (Table 4.4). The questions asked the respondents to rate their personal strength and personal health levels compared with those of their peers.

Approximately 57.8% of all users believed their strength was *above average*, whereas only 27.8% of the nonusers were so inclined ($p<.001$). However, there was a significant difference ($p<.05$) between users and nonusers relative to their intentions to participate in school-sponsored sports in the next academic year (Table 4.3). We can hypothesize that users are more likely to be athletes and therefore believe that their strength is greater than average. In fact, 65.4% of the users who intended to participate in school-sponsored sports thought their strength was above average, whereas only 35.1% of the nonusers who intended to participate in school-sponsored sports responded in the same fashion ($p<.001$). Likewise, 39.7%

Table 4.2 Demographic Data for Anabolic Steroid Users vs. Nonusers

	Respondents (%)	
Characteristic	Users	Nonusers
*Age (years)**		
< 17	7.5	6.2
17	51.8	69.0
18	30.5	23.3
19	4.4	1.4
≥ 20	5.8	0.1
*Race**		
White	77.4	87.8
Black	8.8	4.7
Hispanic	4.9	3.5
Asian	4.0	2.7
Other	4.9	1.3
*Parents' education**		
Not a high school graduate	10.2	5.3
High school graduate	14.2	22.5
Some college	17.7	19.3
College graduate	52.2	49.1
Not known	5.7	3.8

Note. Reprinted from Buckley et al. (1988) by permission.
*$p < .001$.

Table 4.3 School-Sponsored Sport Participation by Anabolic Steroid Use

	Respondents (%)	
Sports participation	Users	Nonusers
*School-sponsored sports participation?**		
Yes	64.8	57.8
No	35.2	42.2
*Main sport at school***		
Baseball or basketball	14.7	21.3
Football	43.5	32.6
Track and field	12.3	14.9
Wrestling	17.2	8.9
Other	12.3	22.3

Note. Reprinted from Buckley et al. (1988) by permission.
*$p < .05$. **$p < .001$.

Table 4.4   **Attitudes and Perceptions of Anabolic Steroid Users and Nonusers**

	Respondents (%)	
Perception	Users	Nonusers
*Strength self-perception**		
Above average	57.8	27.8
Average	31.2	59.2
Below average	6.0	8.8
Don't know	5.0	4.2
*Health self-perception**		
Excellent	39.7	24.1
Very good	31.7	40.7
Good	17.4	29.4
Fair	6.3	5.3
Poor	4.9	0.5

Note. Reprinted from Buckley et al. (1988) by permisson.

*$p < .001$.

of all users reported their overall health as *excellent* compared with only 24.1% of the nonusers ($p<.001$) (Table 4.4). However, perhaps a preexisting bias toward this response was in effect, as previously noted, because 45.9% of the users who intended to participate in school-sponsored sports reported this response, and 29.6% of the nonusers who anticipated participation in sports chose the *excellent* response category ($p<.001$). Interestingly, 4.9% of the users rated their health in the *poor* category versus only 0.5% of the nonusers.

User Characteristics

This study also established a profile of adolescent steroid users. More than one-third of the sample of users (38.3%) reported that they first used anabolic steroids at age 15 years or younger, and another third had started by age 16 years (Figure 4.1). These data indicate that steroids have been used at all high school grade levels and perhaps at the junior high school level as well.

The self-identified users in this study reported from one to more than five cycles of steroid use, with each cycle usually lasting 6 to 12 weeks. Only 18.2% of the users reported one cycle, whereas almost 40% of the users reported five or more cycles of use. Of those who reported first using anabolic steroids at age 15 years or younger, only 9.5% said they had used

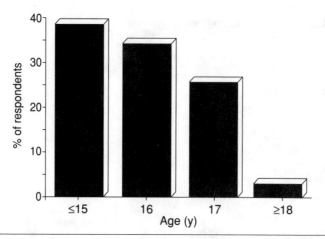

Figure 4.1 Age of respondents at first use of anabolic steroids. *Note.* Reprinted from Buckley et al. (1988) by permission.

the drugs for only one cycle. Twelve percent of the users reported cycles of steroid use lasting 13 weeks or more. A long-term use pattern for some of the users can be postulated even at this early stage of drug abuse.

Approximately 44% of the users said they had used more than one anabolic steroid at the same time (stacking). More revealing is that 38.1% of the users had used both oral and injectable drugs.

The largest percentage of users (47.1%) reported that their main reason for using the drug was *to improve athletic performance* (Figure 4.2). *Appearance* was selected as the main reason for use among 26.7% of the user group. The use of anabolic steroids for injury prevention or treatment, although not a generally accepted medical practice in the United States, was reported by 10.7% of users.

The reported sources of anabolic steroids for this user group included the black market (60.5%), defined as "other athletes, coaches, gyms, etc." (Figure 4.3). However, approximately one-fifth of the users reported that their primary sources were health care professionals (defined in this study as physicians, pharmacists, or veterinarians). Health professionals were the most frequent sources (43%) when the reported reason for steroid use was *to prevent or treat a sports-related injury* versus reasons such as *appearance* (15.5%) and *to increase performance* (18%).

Discussion

This study offers a picture of the nature and scope of anabolic steroid use, information that health professionals can employ when developing intervention strategies, substance control programs, and health risk assessments. Not surprising is the fact that we observed significant variability

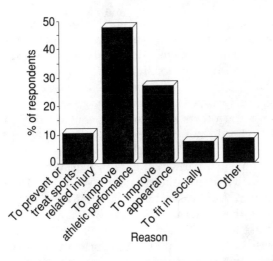

Figure 4.2 Main reasons for using anabolic steroids. *Note.* Reprinted from Buckley et al. (1988) by permission.

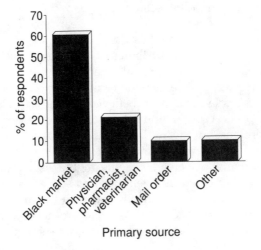

Figure 4.3 Primary sources of anabolic steroids. *Note.* Reprinted from Buckley et al. (1988) by permission.

in user rates among the participating schools, with 15% of the schools having no reported users. This can indicate that drug use is still diffusing, which is in part supported by our finding that schools with small enrollments reported somewhat lower use rates.

The basic user characteristics identified in this study and in the studies reviewed in chapter 3 demonstrate that educational intervention strategies should probably be in place at the junior high school level or earlier. Evidence indicates that adults who deal directly with adolescents need to be aware of user behavior characteristics so that appropriate interventions can be initiated. Such adults obviously include coaches and athletic trainers, but the responsibility can legitimately be broadened to include high school health instructors, physical education specialists, school nurses, school physicians, and others who come in contact with the subgroup of users (35.2%) who do not participate in school-sponsored athletics. Although many of the users in this subgroup may still participate in athletic competition, such participation is primarily on an amateur and individual basis, such as bodybuilding and power lifting. These users may belong to private fitness or health clubs or local YMCAs, or they may train on their own. Still, these data indicate that we may significantly reduce anabolic steroid use by targeting intervention efforts at school-based athletics. In fact, with 43.5% of steroid users reporting participation in interscholastic football, athletic directors, team physicians, coaches, and athletic trainers cannot assume that their institutions are not affected. Also, these data implicate a range of sport activities—such as wrestling, basketball, and track and field—that we cannot overlook in assessing the presence of steroid use at any individual school.

This study elicited descriptive data that researchers can use to establish guidelines for subsequent studies dealing with specific psychological, sociological, or pathological attributes of the anabolic steroid user. The users were more extreme in their health perceptions; the majority believed they were in decidedly better general health than their peers. Similarly, a greater percentage of steroid users believed their strength levels exceeded those of their peers. We cannot use this study to determine the accuracy of these perceptions, but the implication that steroid users perceive benefits from drug use behavior is important. Changing a behavior that has resulted in strongly perceived benefits to the user requires carefully planned and implemented interventions and strategies.

Although we could not specifically establish the prevalence of use at each junior high school grade level, the data strongly indicate significant steroid use by boys 15 years old and younger (38.3%, the largest single response group). This is particularly distressing, because premature epiphyseal closure is potentially a permanent side effect of anabolic steroid use in adolescents. Also, exogenous testosterone and its derivatives have a marked effect on the pituitary gland and testes, resulting in decreased endogenous hormone production and suppression of spermatogenesis. We know that discontinuation of steroid use by mature males results in an eventual return to normal hormonal activity (Strauss, 1987; Swerdloff et al., 1978). This has not been established in biologically immature males, however, and questions remain regarding the effects of anabolic steroid use on pubarche. Anabolic steroids may affect not only the rate of maturation but also the developmental blueprint for biochemical homeostasis.

Coinciding with the evidence of a relatively early onset of steroid use is evidence of what may be described as long-term use behavior. Twelve percent of users in this study reported average cycles of 13 weeks or more. Other studies indicate that adult power lifters who are familiar with steroid use seldom exceed a 13-week cycle (Burkett & Falduto, 1984; Yesalis, Herrick, Buckley, Friedl, Brannon, & Wright, 1988). These adolescents are experimenting with cycle lengths that are longer than those of older steroid users. Long-term use behavior must be further investigated relative to dosage patterns and multiple drug administrations. When one considers that 44% of the users had taken multiple kinds of steroids simultaneously and over 38% had used injectable preparations, it is clear that the potential for the development of long-term use patterns is real.

Prevention

The question becomes, What can the sports community do to change anabolic steroid misuse in the school-age population? Yesalis and Wright (see chapter 14) have outlined three broad areas that may ameliorate the problem:

- interdiction,
- education, and
- alteration of societal values associated with sport and appearance.

Yesalis and Wright outline several demonstrable activities in each of these areas but do not fully comment on how much confidence we can place in these initiatives. Indeed, it is extremely difficult to assess the effectiveness of individual intervention initiatives because the activities involved often overlap strict functional delineations. For example, at the federal level of authority, the Drug Enforcement Administration (DEA) plays an obvious role in interdiction activities related to anabolic steroid use but also has established a nationwide educational effort as part of the demand reduction initiative mandated by the federal charge of the DEA. Although dual roles on the part of interested parties are not necessarily problematic, such roles do make effective coordination with other federal, state, and local enforcement and educational agencies increasingly difficult. It may be a more practical strategy to maintain discrete categorical areas of intervention activities.

Lofquist (1983) defined prevention as the active, assertive process of creating conditions and/or personal attributes that promote well-being. The notion is to promote the well-being of individuals by changing or influencing the conditions under which behaviors exist. Theoretically, the change in conditions promotes acceptable behavior and/or dissuades unacceptable behavior. These changes may occur on a personal level, a societal level, or both. On the personal level, individuals are challenged to clarify their values, knowledge base, attitudes, behavioral intent, and manifest actions. On the societal level, groups of people such as parents, coaches, and athletic administrators are challenged to examine similar criteria.

The objective is to develop a comprehensive prevention program as outlined by Lofquist (1983) that is effective over the three functional areas of intervention (interdiction, education, and societal values) outlined by Yesalis and Wright (chapter 14). A program that deals with anabolic steroid abuse in the high school population should initially focus on the development of the behavior change process as the ultimate goal. The behavior change process should not be limited to adolescents but needs to include parents, coaches, and others who play major roles in influencing the adolescent's attitudes and values related to the importance of winning and appearance.

With this goal in mind, a prevention specialist can develop specific activities within the discrete functional areas of intervention. Following are several assumptions or beliefs that should provide the fundamental bases for the development and implementation of a comprehensive prevention program.

- Individuals (i.e., adolescents, parents, or coaches) are, or can become, responsible for influencing their own environments.
- Internal motivation for change or control over one's circumstances is the most powerful personal resource for effecting change.
- Individual participation in the prevention program development influences compliance.
- The use of existing human and physical resources is preferred to identifying and acquiring new resources.

National Level

Comprehensive prevention programming has been established to deal with drug and alcohol behaviors of the nation's youth. Similarly, large-scale prevention programs addressing health problems such as AIDS, cancer, and heart illness are established and have been proven effective. A preliminary effort in addressing the nonmedical use of anabolic steroids has been reported by the Interagency Task Force on Anabolic Steroids (1991). The Prevention/Education Subcommittee of the task force specifically addressed the development of a strategy for prevention and education related to anabolic steroid abuse and evaluated the effectiveness of education/prevention programs already in place. Essentially, the task force concluded that a lack of general research about anabolic steroids inhibits the development of the content area on which an education effort can be based. The subcommittee also recommended a coordinated federal effort involving the FDA, the National Institute on Drug Abuse, the Office of Substance Abuse Prevention, the Department of Education, and others in implementing a prevention program within 3 to 5 years. Although this report is laudable regarding the education element of prevention programming, it does not represent a call for a truly comprehensive prevention program.

Specific actions to overcome the current lack of a comprehensive prevention program do not need to be particularly novel. A modest effort to fund relevant research, particularly studies related to the physical and psychological effects of the drugs (Yesalis, Wright, & Bahrke, 1989), would help establish the content area and provide a sound basis for legitimate educational efforts. In addition, student athletes can form local groups modeled after the Students Against Drunk Driving (SADD). Local chapters such as these can be established across the country to use the power of positive peer pressure to prevent anabolic steroid use.

Local Level

Cooperation among the network of individuals who are involved in school-based sport activities is paramount, and communication between these different groups or individuals is critical. School superintendents and principals must clearly recognize that the sponsored sport setting requires the same amount of attention as any other sphere of activity under their control. School boards can send this message to administrators by establishing district-wide policy regarding drug prevention activities.

One policy, for example, should relate to the detection or identification of anabolic steroid misuse. Drug use can be identified through drug-testing procedures, self-referral by students at risk, or referrals by concerned adults.

Parents, teachers, coaches, and school officials should be made aware of the signs and symptoms associated with anabolic steroid use, for example, secretive behavior, mood swings, sudden and dramatic weight gain (especially lean mass gain), edema, or gynecomastia (Crawshaw, 1985). In addition, unfamiliar pills and paraphernalia such as vials and needles in an adolescent's possession should raise suspicion.

Drug testing is controversial (Deivert, 1991; Panton, 1989) and involves constitutional issues that revolve around

- the Fourth Amendment clause prohibiting unreasonable search and seizures;
- the Fourteenth Amendment's due-process clause, which protects property interests created and defined by state law;
- the elements of the Fifth Amendment's protection against self-incrimination; and

- the Ninth and Fourteenth Amendments' elements of personal liberty and reservation of rights, respectively, which are generally recognized as support clauses for the generic concept of the right of privacy (Brock & McKenna, 1988; Cochran, 1988; Partridge, 1989).

Although opinions vary somewhat, defensible drug testing programs for anabolic steroids have been established at the high school level and sponsored by the athletic programs (Thurston, 1990). However, although efficiencies of scale and technology have allowed for high schools to implement drug-testing programs in general, the cost of drug tests for anabolic steroids, relative to costs for other illicit drugs, is prohibitive for most secondary schools (see chapter 13).

In developing policy on steroid use we must direct particular attention at clearly outlining procedural detail and effective sanctions. The athletic director should take a leadership role by clearly establishing athletic department policy. The athletic director can define procedures for the various groups of individuals within his or her sphere of influence. Procedures can include

- identification and referral procedures for coaching and support staff;
- evaluation and implementation of sanction procedures that relate specifically to the athletic department;
- education requirements for athletes, coaches, parents, and support staff; and
- procedural oversight of medical care delivery.

Coaches can dovetail appropriate team policy and procedures regarding the comprehensive drug prevention program with athletic department and district initiatives. Activities conducted by the coach are critical because they are the operative interface between the athletic program and the participants. Observation as a drug-use identification mechanism can be most effectively carried out by the coaching staff. The frequent contact between the coach and the participants provides for unequaled opportunities for content education, values clarification, and development of coping strategies to deal with difficult or adverse situations. Likewise, the team physician, athletic trainer, or school nurse is in an excellent position to identify adolescents at risk of steroid use.

Similarly, teachers are in a position to recognize students who abuse steroids because of changes in physical appearance or behavior that can be observed in the classroom. Furthermore teachers, in general, are trained as effective conduits of information. Health teachers are specifically trained to reinforce content presentation with specific models for promoting behavioral change among students.

Obviously, education is one of the key items in a comprehensive drug abuse prevention program. However, the educational process is itself multifaceted and if approached in a disjointed fashion is destined to be ineffective. Unfortunately, many people view the sum total of the education process as the presentation of information. If behavioral change is the measure or criteria of success, the transfer of information is a small part of an effective package. Other components involve behavioral intent, behavioral modification, and affective criteria. A single-session content-oriented education initiative has been found to be severely lacking as an effective intervention strategy for steroid abuse (Carlson et al., 1991; Goldberg et al., 1991). On the other hand, Bents and co-workers (1990) found that an education program that emphasized alternatives to anabolic steroid use, such as nutrition principles and strength-training techniques, was more effective in improving attitudes toward potential anabolic steroid use than either an education program in which no alternatives were discussed or no intervention program. Furthermore, Goldberg et al. (1991) found that an anabolic steroid education program that emphasized only the negative consequences ("scare tactics") of anabolic steroids was ineffective. Yet another report (Frankle & Lefters, 1990) suggested that education alone may not be as effective as clinical assessment and consultation for individuals who abuse steroids.

Conclusion

This study has established the presence of anabolic steroid use among high school males. Based on our findings, 6.6% of 12th-grade male students use or have used these drugs. More importantly, if the steroid use rate from our sample is applied to the national population of males enrolled in secondary schools, it suggests that between 250,000 and 500,000 adolescents in the country have used or are currently using steroids. Consequently, at both the national and local levels comprehensive and coordinated prevention programs need to be implemented that openly recognize the role our society has played in creating the demand for these drugs.

References

Bents, R., Young, J., Bosworth, E., Boyea, S., Elliott, D., & Goldberg, L. (1990). An effective educational program alters attitudes toward anabolic steroid use among adolescent athletes. *Medicine and Science in Sports and Exercise, 22*(2), S64.

Brock, S.F., & McKenna, K.M. (1988). Drug testing in sport. *Dickinson Law Review*, Spring, *92*, 505-567.

Buckley, W.E., Yesalis, C.E., Friedl, K.E., Anderson, W.A., Streit, A.L., & Wright, J.E. (1988). Estimated prevalence of anabolic steroid use among male high school seniors. *Journal of the American Medical Association, 260*(23), 3441-3445.

Burkett, L.N., & Falduto, M.T. (1984). Steroid use by athletes in a metropolitan area. *The Physician and Sportsmedicine, 12*, 69-74.

Carlson, N., Cleary, B., Thompson, H.R., Bents, R., Folker, R., Elliot, D., & Goldberg, L. (1991). Attitudes after teaching to deter anabolic steroid use: How durable are the drugs? *Medicine and Science in Sports and Exercise*, **23**(Suppl. 4), 558.

Cochran, J.O. (1988). Drug testing of athletes and the United States Constitution: Crisis and conflict. *Dickinson Law Review*, Spring 92, **82**, 571-607.

Crawshaw, J. (1985, August 15). Recognizing anabolic steroid abuse. *Patient Care*, pp. 28-47.

Deivert, R.G. (1991). The role of the Constitution in the drug testing of student-athletes in the public schools. *Journal of Alcohol and Drug Education*, **36**(2), 32-41.

English, G. (1987). A theoretical explanation of why athletes choose to use steroids, and the role of the coach in influencing behavior. *National Strength Conditioning Association Journal*, **9**, 53-56.

Frankle, M., & Lefters, D. (1990). Hooked on hormones. *Journal of the American Medical Association*, **263**, 2049.

Goldberg, L., Bents, R., Bosworth, E., Trevisan, L., & Elliot, D. (1991). Anabolic steroid education and adolescents: Do scare tactics work? *Pediatrics*, **87**(3), 283-286.

Interagency Task Force on Anabolic Steroids Report. (1991, January). Washington, DC: U.S. Department of Health and Human Services, Public Health Service.

Jessor, R. (1982). Problem behavior and developmental transition in adolescence. *Journal of School Health*, **52**, 295-300.

Lofquist, W. (1983). *Discovering the meaning of prevention*. Tucson, AZ: Ayd.

Panton, S. (1989, April). Drug testing: Exploring legal rights of student-athletes. *Athletic Administration*, pp. 13-15.

Partridge, L.R. (1989). Making the grade: Can student drug testing programs in public schools pass a legal challenge? *Willamette Law Review*, **25**(165), 165-196.

Powell, J. (1987). 636,000 Injuries annually in high school football. *Athletic Training*, **22**, 19-22.

Strauss, R.H. (1987). Anabolic steroids. In R.H. Strauss (Ed.), *Drugs and performance in sports* (pp. 59-67). Philadelphia: Saunders.

Swerdloff, R.S., Palacios, A., Anselmo, P., McClure, R.D., Campfield, L., & Browman, S. (1978). Male contraception: Clinical assessment of chronic administration of testosterone enanthate. *International Journal of Andrology*, April (Suppl. 2), 731-747.

Thurston, J. (1990). Chemical warfare: Battling steroids in athletes. *Marquette Sports Law Journal*, **1**(93), 93-143.

Whiting-O'Keefe, Q.E., Henke, C., & Simborg, D.W. (1984). Choosing the correct unit of analysis in medical care experiments. *Medical Care*, **22**, 1101-1114.

Yesalis, C., Herrick, R., Buckley, W., Friedl, K.E., Brannon, D., & Wright, J.E. (1988). Self-reported use of anabolic-androgenic steroids by elite power lifters. *The Physician and Sportsmedicine*, **16**, 91-100.

Yesalis, C., Wright, J., & Bahrke, M. (1989). Epidemiology and policy issues in the measurement of the long term effects of anabolic-androgenic steroids. *Sports Medicine*, **8**, 129-138.

PART II

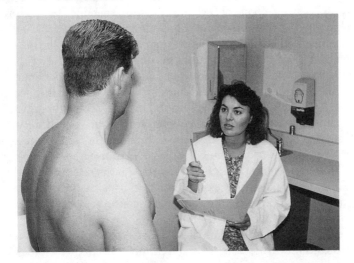

Effects, Dependence, and Treatment Issues

The background information learned in Part I allows us to now turn our attention to the physical and psychological effects of anabolic steroids as well as to issues of clinical assessment and treatment.

In chapter 5, John Lombardo attempts to answer the question, Do anabolic steroids enhance athletic performance? To do so, he describes the multifaceted nature of athletic performance, listing the many factors that can determine success in sport, and presents the results of studies that assess the ergogenic effects of anabolic steroids. Lastly, he discusses the differences in the results of the studies reviewed and a number of mechanisms that have been proposed to explain the actions of anabolic steroids on muscular strength and lean body mass.

Adverse physical effects of anabolic steroids are discussed in chapters 6 and 7. Although chapter 6 concentrates on the adverse effects that are produced in normally virilized men by exogenous androgens or by pharmacological properties of the modified anabolic steroids, many of these effects apply to women as well. Chapter 7 then focuses on the effects of anabolic steroids specific to females. Additional information on patterns of use, drugs used, and reasons for use is included as well.

In chapter 8, we shift our attention to psychological effects. Michael Bahrke discusses potential mechanisms for some androgen effects on the nervous system, the relationship between endogenous testosterone levels and aggression, the effects of the clinical use of anabolic steroids on mood and behavior, the relationship of anabolic steroid use to mental health, and the major methodological issues involved in assessing the relationship between androgen levels and mood and behavior.

Chapter 9 reviews what we know about the potential of anabolic steroids to produce dependence and highlights areas for further study. The author defines *drug dependence* clinically and scientifically and discusses mechanisms, predictors, and the course of anabolic steroid dependence.

The authors of chapter 10 review data from the study presented in chapter 4 in relation to psychological aspects of use and the potential for dependence to develop. This chapter examines the relationships between dependence potential and age of initiation of use; frequency of use; methods of administration; unwillingness to discontinue use; and perceptions of strength, health, and peer use.

Having looked at issues of physical and psychological dependence, we now focus on clinical assessment and treatment. In chapter 11, Kirk Brower explains the processes of identifying the steroid user in the clinical setting, assessing (or evaluating) that user, and treating the ex-user who may suffer symptoms of withdrawal.

CHAPTER 5

The Efficacy and Mechanisms of Action of Anabolic Steroids

John Lombardo

In spite of the claims made by some of the investigators that the use of anabolic steroids by male athletes in conjunction with progressive weight resistance training will afford a greater increase in lean muscle bulk and greater strength than by weight resistance training alone, there is, in fact, no substantial evidence that this is so.

ALLAN J. RYAN
Federation Proceedings, 1981 (**40**)

Portions of this chapter are from Lombardo (1990) and reprinted from Lombardo, Hickson, and Lamb (1991) by permission; see credits page for more information.

Do anabolic steroids enhance athletic performance? To answer this question, we must understand the multifaceted nature of athletic performance. Rarely, if ever, does a solitary factor determine success in sport; rather, success is a result of optimal development of many factors (from Lombardo, 1987, used by permission):

Level of conditioning—Conditioning includes strength, flexibility, muscular endurance, and cardiovascular endurance. The relative importance of each of these differs depending upon the sport or event.

Skill—Development of skill is a learned behavior based on genetic predisposition and repetition (practice). Some sport successes rely only on the development of gross motor skills. However, other sports require fine and complex motor skill development.

Diet—An athlete's diet provides the fuel that the athlete needs to perform. Until recently the athletic population has neglected nutrition. The fund of knowledge in this area is rapidly expanding, and the role of diet is increasing as the field of sport nutrition develops.

Psyche—The athlete's mind set, mental, or psychological state is described by phrases such as "getting up for a game," "raising the intensity level," and "game face on." These terms have long been part of sports. As the field of psychology has been applied to sports, new phrases such as "focus," "visualization," and "relaxation" have been added to sport jargon.

Opponent—The opponent's style of play, strengths, and weaknesses (commonly referred to as *matchups*) affect one's performance and success.

Arena—The home-field advantage appears to be a real phenomenon. It may be the influence of the spectators, familiarity with the environment, maintenance of daily routine, or a combination of these and other factors, which give the home team an edge.

Sleep—Proper rest is important in the performance of any task, especially when complex motor skills are involved. Because of pre-event anxiety, a new environment, or the circuslike atmosphere that sometimes surrounds certain events, athletes may have difficulty sleeping.

Genes—This is arguably the most important factor and one over which the athlete has absolutely no control. Many of the characteristics that are key to success in sports are results of these genetic expressions, which have been referred to as "natural ability" and "raw talent."

Drugs—Drugs can have two effects. The performance of an athlete who abuses illicit drugs such as cocaine or marijuana or the legal drug alcohol can be adversely affected. Performance-enhancing drugs, such as anabolic steroids, are used to improve performance and potentially make a difference in the outcome of the competition.

In events in which centimeters or milliseconds are the difference between success and failure, how much does manipulation of one factor contribute? When 20 to 30 lb of lean mass can make the difference between a lucrative professional contract (with the accompanying adulation and fame) and the pay and routine of most other jobs, how many athletes will use anabolic steroids to reach their goals?

Individuals who use anabolic steroids desire benefits such as

- alteration of body composition (increased lean mass and reduced fat),
- increased strength,
- increased endurance,
- hastened recovery from exercise (i.e., ability to perform longer, more frequent, and/or higher intensity workouts), and
- enhanced athletic performance.

Do anabolic steroids give the desired benefits? To answer the question we can turn to two sources of information: the scientific literature, which includes studies of both animals and humans, and the consistent but perhaps questionable anecdotal evidence given by athletes and other users (Starr, 1981). Although it is important to base one's knowledge as a scientist on accurate data derived from well-designed experiments, one should never completely ignore the results of case reports and anecdotal evidence.

Animal Studies

The results of animal studies regarding the use of anabolic steroids are consistent. Normal male animals who are exercised have consistently shown no increase in body weight or improvement in performance after anabolic steroid treatment (Hickson et al., 1976; Richardson, 1977; Young, Crookshank, & Ponder, 1977). The problems with applying these results to humans are the differences in types of exercise (running on a treadmill and swimming for animals vs. progressive resistance exercise for humans) and the uncertainty as to whether the psychological effects of the human's competitive drive can be simulated in the animal.

However, castrated male rats (Heitzman, 1976; Kochakian & Endahl, 1959), normal female rats (Exner, Staudte, & Pette, 1973; Heitzman, 1976; Hervey & Hutchinson, 1973), and cattle and poultry (Nesheim, 1976) have consistently exhibited significant increases in nitrogen retention and lean body mass after steroid treatment. These increases in nitrogen retention and lean mass occurred whether or not the animals exercised.

Human Studies

The literature on the effects of anabolic steroids on lean body mass, strength, and aerobic capacity in humans is contradictory and confusing. As one reviews these studies perhaps some clarity can emerge.

Aerobic Capacity and Endurance

Because anabolic steroids stimulate bone marrow to produce red blood cells (erythropoiesis), it has been hypothesized that steroid administration can increase the oxygen-carrying capacity of the blood and thereby improve maximal oxygen uptake ($\dot{V}O_2$max), a measure of aerobic capacity, which is calculated using indirect measures. If steroid use does bring about an increase in maximal oxygen uptake, an increase in aerobic endurance performance should follow. Studies have reported increases in this indirect measure of aerobic capacity ($\dot{V}O_2$max) in men at various levels of aerobic conditioning who were administered steroids (Albrecht & Albrecht, 1969; Johnson & O'Shea, 1969; Keul, Deus, & Kinderman, 1976). But there also have been reports of no increase in aerobic capacity with steroid use in similar circumstances (Fahey & Brown, 1973; Hervey et al., 1976; Johnson, Fisher, Silvester, & Hofheins, 1972; Johnson, Roundy, Allsen, Fisher, & Silvester, 1975). These contradictory results raise some interesting questions.

- Is the $\dot{V}O_2$max, which was used in these studies, an accurate indicator of success in endurance events?
- Is the $\dot{V}O_2$max measurement sensitive enough to record changes that will be significant in the results of an endurance event?

Because tests of $\dot{V}O_2$max (and especially tests that do not directly measure $\dot{V}O_2$max) are not necessarily good predictors of endurance performance (Saltin & Åstrand, 1967), it is unclear what effect steroid use has on such performance. Consequently, it would be interesting to observe the effects of steroids on a direct measure of aerobic endurance performance. Furthermore, because the effect of steroids on red blood cell production in normal men is relatively small, there is only a weak rationale for hypothesizing a beneficial effect of steroids on endurance performance.

However, endurance athletes might benefit from steroids if the athletes were able to perform more frequent, longer, high-intensity workouts as a result of steroid use. The performance advantage an athlete will incur through such an increase in workouts is pure conjecture at this time. However, because the ability to perform these frequent high-intensity workouts is the rationale for steroid use given by endurance runners (Wright, personal communication, Sept. 5, 1989; Yesalis, personal communication, 1990), this is certainly an area in which investigation is warranted. Until such investigations are conducted, questions concerning the effect of anabolic steroids on performance in endurance events will remain unanswered.

Body Composition

The users of anabolic steroids believe that in conjunction with training, steroid use will increase their lean body mass and decrease their fat mass. Does the scientific literature support these beliefs? A number of training studies have shown no significant increase in lean body mass with the use of anabolic steroids, whereas other studies have shown significant increases (Table 5.1).

Griggs et al. (1989), using pharmacologic doses of testosterone enanthate (3 mg/kg/week), reported significant increases in muscle protein synthesis in normal nonexercising men. However, the authors found no significant increase in muscle fiber diameter despite significant increases in weight. Crist, Stackpole, and Peake (1983) studied the effects of a low dose of steroids administered for 3 weeks, on the body composition of experienced weight trainers who consumed supplemental protein; the authors used underwater weighing and found no increase in lean body mass. Hervey et al. (1981) studied experienced weight lifters for 6 weeks, using no dietary controls but administering 100 mg methandrosternolone daily. The researchers found significant increases in lean body mass by underwater weighing, skin folds, and anthropometric measurements. Similar increases in lean body mass were found by Hervey et al. (1976) in an earlier study that differed from their later study only in the choice of subjects (physical education majors who were inexperienced weight lifters). Table 5.1 compares these and other studies of the effects of anabolic steroids on lean body mass. Fowler, Gardner, and Egstrom (1965); Fahey and Brown (1973); Golding, Freydinger, and Fishel (1974); Stromme, Meen, and Aakvaag (1974); and Crist et al. (1983) reported no significant changes in lean body mass with the use of anabolic steroids. But O'Shea (1971); Ward (1973); Stamford and Moffatt (1974); Hervey et al. (1976, 1981); Loughton and Ruhling (1977); and Alen, Hakkinen, and Komi (1984) all found significant increases in lean body mass. Interestingly, only Golding et al. (1974) and Crist et al. (1983) found no increases in lean body mass with experienced weight trainers, and only Hervey et al. (1976) found significant lean body mass increases with inexperienced weight lifters.

Table 5.1 **Efficacy of Anabolic Steroids**

Variable	Golding et al. (1974)	Stromme et al. (1974)	Hervey et al. (1981)	Hervey et al. (1976)	Ward (1973)	Fahey & Brown (1973)
Duration (weeks)	12	8	6 (3 times)	6 (3 times)	5	9
Intensity	Mod to Heavy	Mod to Heavy	Mod to Heavy	Mod to Heavy	Heavy	Light to Mod
Frequency (days/week)	4	3	—	—	3?	3
Drug/dosage	? 10 mg ?	Mes 75-100 mg	Met 100 mg	Met 100 mg	Met 10 mg	Nand 1 mg/week
Diet	↑ Prot	↑ Prot	—	—	—	—
Experienced/ inexperienced weight lifter	Exp	Inexp?	Exp	Inexp	Exp	Inexp
Weight/lean body mass	– SF	– Ant	+ UW SF Ant	+ UW SF Ant	+ UW	– UW
Strength	—	—	+	—	+	—

94

Variable	Stamford & Moffatt (1974)	Crist et al. (1983)	Loughton & Ruhling (1977)	Fowler et al. (1965)	O'Shea (1971)	Alen et al. (1984)
Duration (weeks)	8	3 (3 times)	7	16	4	24
Intensity	Heavy	Mod to Heavy	Mod to Heavy	Light	Mod to Heavy	Heavy
Frequency (days/week)	3	—	6	5	3	6
Drug/dosage	Met 10	Nand Test 100 mg/week	Met 10	Met 20	Met 10	Varied
Diet	↑ Prot	↑ Prot	↑ Prot	—	↑ Prot	Adequate Protein
Experienced/inexperienced weight lifter	Exp	Exp	Exp? Inexp	Inexp	Exp	Exp
Weight/lean body mass	+ Ant	- UW	+ BWT	- SF Ant	+ SF	+ SF
Strength	+	-	-	-	+	+

Note. Mod = moderate; Mes = mestoranum; Met = methandrostenolone; Nand = nandrolone; Test = testosterone; Prot = protein; Exp = experienced weight lifter; Inexp = inexperienced weight lifter; SF = skinfolds; Ant = anthropometric; UW = underwater weighing; BWT = body weight; + = positive effect; – = no effect; ↑ = increased; — = no information available; ? = unknown or unclear.

Reprinted from Lombardo (1990).

In summary, there is contradictory evidence in the literature about the effect of anabolic steroids on lean body mass. However, we can conclude that "anabolic/androgenic steroids, in the presence of an adequate diet, can contribute to increases in body weight, often in the lean mass compartment" (ACSM, 1984, p. 13).

Strength Performance

The literature contains more contradictory findings concerning the effects of anabolic steroids on strength training (Table 5.1). Stamford and Moffatt (1974) found significant strength increases in their study of prisoners who were experienced weight trainers and who were given supplemental protein with a low dosage of anabolic steroids. Crist et al. (1983) found no significant increases in strength under similar conditions. The short duration of each treatment period (3 weeks) and the dosage of drug (100 mg nandrolone decanoate/week), which is much less than that used by many strength athletes, are notable criticisms of the study by Crist et al.

About one-half of the research reports have shown no significant increases in strength with the use of anabolic-androgenic steroids (Crist et al., 1983; Fahey & Brown, 1973; Fowler et al., 1965; Golding, 1974; Hervey et al., 1976; Loughton & Ruhling, 1977; Stromme et al., 1974). Other studies have shown significant increases in strength (Alen et al., 1984; Hervey et al., 1981; O'Shea, 1971; Stamford & Moffatt, 1974; Ward, 1973). As a whole, this research does not overwhelmingly support either the presence or absence of an ergogenic effect of anabolic-androgenic steroids on strength.

This contradiction is well illustrated in Table 5.2, which compares two studies by the same laboratory (Hervey et al., 1976, 1981). These similar studies both employed a crossover design with a 6-week treatment of drug or placebo, a 5- or 6-week washout period (time without drug), and a 6-week treatment on the opposite condition (period with drug or placebo).

Both studies used the dosage most closely resembling that used by many of the athletes who abuse anabolic steroids, but the studies still showed differences in the effect of steroids on strength. The major difference between the two studies was the weight-lifting experience of the subjects. Because many variables affect maximal strength performance, it is extremely difficult to detect statistically significant effects of any experimental treatment with a small number of subjects.

Therefore, because many studies do report a positive effect of steroid administration on strength performance, the ACSM (1984) has concluded that "the gains in muscular strength achieved through high intensity exercise and proper diet can be increased by the use of anabolic/androgenic steroids in some individuals" (p. 13).

Table 5.2   Comparison of Hervey's Studies on the Effect of Steroids on Strength Performance

Variable	Hervey et al., 1976	Hervey et al., 1981
Drug (Methandrostenolone)	100 mg/day	100 mg/day
Subjects (N/source)	11 Physical education majors	7 Experienced weight lifters
Body weight	Increased	Increased
Fat-free mass	Increased	Increased
Strength	No significant change	Increased

Note. Reprinted from Lombardo, Hickson, and Lamb (1991) by permission.

Reasons for Differences in Results of Studies

Why are there so many differences in the studies that report the ergogenic effects of androgens? Control of independent variables such as diet, weight-training experience, and drug dosage has been inconsistent in the experimental studies on the ergogenic effects of anabolic steroids. Lamb (1984) concluded that there is no systematic pattern in the variables to explain the differences in steroid effects on strength. However, Wright (1978) and Yesalis, Wright, and Lombardo (1989) proposed a number of potential explanations for the confusing results (Table 5.3).

The following factors deserve special attention:

The weight-training experience of the subject—Many of the studies used inexperienced weight trainers, who are known to make significant early gains when beginning strength training programs. These large gains in strength probably are not significantly increased by anabolic steroids in this early part of the conditioning program. Experienced weight trainers, on the other hand, have plateaued and their gains in strength are smaller as they continue training. In these experienced individuals, drug-assisted increases, which might be small in comparison to the larger gains by the novice lifter, will be significant compared to smaller gains that the experienced lifter can attain solely by training during the 6-week study.

The intensity of training—Many studies utilized low-intensity, short-duration, low-frequency workouts, which are not comparable in terms of physiologic and biochemical effects to the high-intensity, long-duration, high-frequency workouts performed by many athletes who use anabolic steroids.

Table 5.3   Reasons for Lack of Consensus on Anabolic Steroids' Effects on Performance Variables in Human Subjects

Subjects	The number of subjects, their experience in weight training, and their physical condition at the start of the study varied.
Diet	Most not controlled or recorded.
Training methods	Volumes and intensities varied.
Testing methods	Strength often not measured in the training mode. Body compositions often assessed from skinfold estimates.
Drugs	Variable; few studies reported on athletes' self-administering multiple drugs.
Study design	Some crossover, some single blind, some double blind, some not blind, some no controls.
Mechanisms of action	Unknown and varying degrees of anabolic and anticatabolic action, as well as interaction with motivational effects.
Dose	Variable; only two studies administered dosages approximating those currently used by competing strength athletes.
Length of study	Variable and generally short; lack of reports on prolonged training and self-administration of steroids.
Placebo effect	Difficulty in assessment of placebo effect due to easy detection by athletes of steroid administration; consequent lack of blind studies.
Data interpretation	Differing backgrounds (scientific, clinical, athletic, administrative), perspectives, and goals of interpreters.
Legal and ethical issues	Preclude design and execution of well-controlled studies using doses and patterns of administration of drugs with unknown long-term effects in healthy volunteers in a manner comparable to those of many current steroid users.

Note. Reprinted from Yesalis, Wright, and Lombardo (1989) by permission.

Dietary controls—Many of the studies did not control dietary intake. None of the studies reported the amount of calories or the percentage of carbohydrates, protein, and fat in the diets of the subjects. These factors are extremely important when one is measuring lean body mass and strength as the indicators of efficacy of a drug.

Dosage of the drug—Athletes use dosages of anabolic steroids up to 100 times or more of replacement levels; no studies have approached these doses. Ethically, such a study cannot be done, because the long-term health effects of these doses are not known (see chapter 6). Whether the high-dose regimens and multiple-drug regimens commonly used by the athletes are beneficial is unknown.

Specificity of training—Some of the studies used isometric or isokinetic testing as the end points, yet the subjects used isotonic training; this difference between the methods of training and testing surely affects the results.

Women and Children

There have been no studies of the effects of anabolic steroids on strength or body composition of women and children, in whom the use of these drugs has reportedly increased (see chapters 2, 3, 4, and 7). Clinical trials in these two groups pose an ethical problem because of the irrevocable virilizing effects of the drugs (see chapters 6 and 7). However, in view of the effects of androgens demonstrated in animal studies on castrated males (Heitzman, 1976; Kochakian & Endahl, 1959) and on females (Exner et al., 1973; Heitzman, 1976; Hervey & Hurchinson, 1973; Nesheim, 1976), we can expect a positive ergogenic effect in these two groups, who have lower endogenous levels of testosterone than adult males (Kochakian, 1976).

Mechanisms of Action

A number of mechanisms have been proposed to explain the actions of anabolic steroids on muscular strength and lean body mass. These include

- an increase in protein synthesis,
- inhibition of the catabolic effect of glucocorticoids,
- effects on the central nervous system and the neuromuscular junctions, and
- the placebo effect.

Anabolic steroids are called *anabolic* because they increase protein synthesis through their interactions with specific receptors in target tissues that include skeletal and cardiac muscle, skin, testes, prostate, and various areas of the brain. These hormone-receptor complexes interact with the receptor sites on the chromosomes, which elicit gene transcription and the subsequent synthesis of messenger ribonucleic acid (RNA). Various enzymes and contractual and structural proteins are the ultimate result of this process (Kochakian, 1976; Kruskemper, 1968). Rogozkin (1976, 1979) demonstrated that exercise increases the rate of transcription as measured by increased RNA polymerase activity. He also showed that

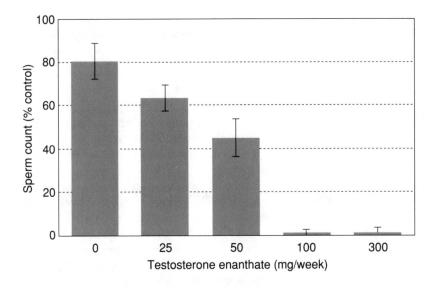

Figure 6.3 Sperm counts, expressed as a proportion of individual baseline values, at different doses of testosterone enanthate administered weekly by intramuscular injection for 6 months. *Note.* Adapted from Matsumoto and Bremner (1988).

(1959) are not those that athletes are generally known to be using; in fact, the closest relative tested was the androgenic progestogen norethandrolone, and this has not been reported to be used by athletes. Finally, none of the authors of this study suggested that the effects might be permanent and no studies since then have made such a suggestion.

Spermatogenic Rebound With Cessation of Steroid Administration

High-dose androgens have also been administered to restore fertility in men with low sperm counts, through a well-recognized but poorly understood rebound that occurs following several months of high-dose androgen sperm suppression (Charney & Gordon, 1978; Rowley & Heller, 1972). Up to 60% of patients with below-normal spermatogenic activity but otherwise normal seminiferous epithelia show at least temporary improvement in their sperm counts, and some patients show permanent improvement. Norethandrolone, testosterone esters, and mesterolone have all been used in rebound therapy, and some researchers claim that these drugs improve pregnancy success rates. Other approaches to treatment of male infertility have included administration of mesterolone

(Aafjes, Van der Vijver, Brugman, & Schenck, 1983) or testosterone undecanoate (Kloer, Hoogen, & Nieschlag, 1980) to oligospermic men in an attempt to support spermatogenesis.

Gonadotropic Relation

The reduction of sperm count is primarily mediated through the suppression of gonadotropins (LH and FSH), although there may be some direct effects on the testes as well. This gonadotropin suppression has been well demonstrated in many of the contraceptive studies as well as in at least one detailed assessment of self-administering athletes (Alen, Rahkila, Reinila, & Vihko, 1987). Earlier studies have suggested that orally active mesterolone does not suppress gonadotropins at doses that elicit androgenic effects (Aakvaag & Stromme, 1974; Petry, Rausch-Stroomann, Hienz, Senge, & Mauss, 1968) and that 17-alkylated androgens also may not suppress gonadotropins at moderate doses (Friedl et al., 1990). Some steroid-using athletes administer human chorionic gonadotropin (HCG) during or at the end of their steroid cycles with the intention of preventing the reduction in activity or restimulating the testes to a more rapid recovery. Some evidence indicates that this will maintain testicular function during steroid use (Wing, Ewing, Zegeye, & Zirkin, 1985), but this may require more careful dosing than self-medicating athletes are likely to achieve. The testes were not fully responsive to a single dose of HCG in athletes treated 3 weeks after the ends of their cycles of steroid use (Martikainen, Alen, Rahkila, & Vihko, 1986), whereas repeated HCG treatments actually desensitized the testes to LH stimulation (Glass & Vigersky, 1980). The main risk that athletes run in this use of HCG is an increased probability for the development of gynecomastia (Freidl & Yesalis, 1989).

Binding Protein Effects

Sex hormone-binding globulin (SHBG) is reduced by both 17-alkylated androgens and the esters (Friedl et al., 1991), but the 17-alkylated androgens are more potent in this effect (Friedl et al., 1990), reflecting either the difference in androgen/estrogen balance produced with these two classes of androgens or the difference in direct hepatic actions of these pharmacological preparations. SHBG is also reduced in steroid-using athletes (Ruokonen, Alen, Bolton, & Vihko, 1985), which leads to an increase in free and albumin-bound testosterone. The significance of this change is uncertain because many of the synthetic androgens have a reduced binding affinity to begin with (Saartok, Dahlberg, & Gustafsson, 1984) and will be little affected; however, we can predict that a diminished SHBG level will result in a higher clearance rate for testosterone and other steroids that are bound by SHBG.

Case Reports of Athlete Users

One report in the orthopedic literature describes two case reports of athletes who, the report claims, demonstrate sustained hypogonadism as a result of their steroid use (Jarow & Lipshultz, 1990). This report demonstrates some of the problems encountered with such uncontrolled "studies." One bodybuilder had used androgens off and on for 4 years and was using high doses of three different androgens until 6 weeks before his work-up for infertility, when he demonstrated a low sperm count, reduced testosterone concentration, and poor response to gonadotropin releasing hormone (GnRH) stimulation. One year later he still demonstrated a poor response to GnRH stimulation; however, the report did not verify that he had discontinued his steroid use. This is important, because I have encountered a similar case in which the husband was willing to let his wife go through a complete series of infertility tests before he would admit that he was still using anabolic steroids (Friedl, 1987). The second case cited by Jarow and Lipshultz (1990) was a 39-year-old competitive weight lifter who had fathered three children and now complained of decreased libido; he also had a history of epididymitis. He was found to have a reduced testosterone concentration but normal gonadotropin levels, and one semen analysis was within normal ranges. The report provided no details about this patient's treatment including whether or not he received a prescription for steroids. The authors reported these two cases to highlight "the potentially permanent deleterious effects of anabolic steroids to the hypothalamic-pituitary-gonadal axis" (p. 431). These case reports illustrate several key problems that recur in this case report literature. The cessation of steroid use was not verified, the pre-steroid-use clinical status was unknown, and the clinical testing was inadequate for any conclusive diagnosis.

Conclusions

From the evidence of studies of androgen administration, it is not readily apparent that we can attribute significant adverse health effects to androgens as a general class; however, the 17-alkyl-substituted androgens have certain established consequences, all involving the liver. The 17-alkylated androgens produce a consistent and substantial reduction in HDLC/LDLC fractions, possibly increasing the risk of heart disease, although this outcome remains to be demonstrated in androgen users. Cholestatic jaundice has been observed in frequencies ranging from none to 17% in various categories of patients treated with 17-alkylated androgen, but this condition is readily reversed when androgen treatment is stopped. Peliosis hepatis is clearly associated with use of 17-alkylated androgen but with unknown frequency. Hepatic tumors are rare in men but occur with a frequency as high as 1 to 3% with 17-alkylated androgen treatment, with a latency of 2 to 30 years. Nearly half of these discovered tumors rupture, although a larger proportion of benign disease may remain undetected. In two cases, including one of a self-medicating bodybuilder, rupture proved fatal.

In contrast to the orally active androgens, androgen esters produce few reports of adverse effects, even though the clinical use of these injected androgens appears to be widespread. This is the basis for their use in male contraceptive trials (World Health Organization Task Force, 1990). However, several case reports involving death or significant illness in athletes self-administering androgens suggest the possibility of other adverse effects that have not been commonly associated with androgen doses in the clinical range. Foremost among these reports are the three cases of stroke reported in bodybuilders and a fourth in a hypogonadal man, who self-administered high doses of androgen. Because there is no established steroid dosing that can be recommended to produce desired competitive advantages of increased strength or increased aggressiveness, athletes use doses and steroids with no defined upper limit. This is substantially different from the approach used in the development of male steroidal contraception, for which the lowest effective dose has been carefully determined (Matsumoto, 1990). We may speculate that more serious side effects such as thrombotic stroke occur at very high doses, even with androgen esters, through estrogenic metabolites or by crossover interactions with nonandrogenic receptors. Researchers have speculated that suppression of immune function is a possible consequence through crossover interaction with corticosteroid receptors, although the only study that has examined immune function in androgen-using athletes found an enhancement of immune function (primarily enhanced natural killer-cell activity) in the steroid users (Calabrese et al., 1989). These higher dose effects may only become apparent with prospective study of androgen abusers, that group with no scientifically determined steroid dosing rationale and, especially, with no dose upper limit. Based on case reports of adverse effects, this group may comprise primarily bodybuilders.

Clearly, 17-alkyl substitution in an androgen introduces properties producing health risks that should not be ascribed to androgenic actions, and other nonandrogenic health consequences will occur through the use of black-market preparations of uncertain quality and composition. Other distinctions are emerging even between androgen esters (Friedl et al., 1991; Hannan et al., 1991; Hobbs et al., 1991), which suggest that testosterone esters, indistinguishable from endogenous testosterone after the compounds are hydrolyzed in circulation, are potent androgens possessing the fewest short-term health risks at high doses of up to 300 mg/week for at least several months. On the other hand, there is reasonable suspicion that prostatic carcinoma is linked to androgen excess (Ross et al., 1986;

Schally & Comaru-Schally, 1987). The bottom line is that an athlete would be foolish to conclude that there is a safe way to use anabolic steroids; although no disease of androgen excess has ever been described for men, the long-term consequences of androgen supplementation have not been investigated and are simply unknown.

References

Aakvaag, A., & Stromme, S.B. (1974). The effect of mesterolone administration to normal men on the pituitary-testicular function. *Acta Endocrinologica*, **77**, 380-386.

Adamson, J.W., & Vapnek, D. (1991). Recombinant erythropoeitin to improve athletic performance. *New England Journal of Medicine*, **324**, 698-699.

Aiache, A.E. (1989). Surgical treatment of gynecomastia in the body builder. *Plastic and Reconstructive Surgery*, **83**, 61-66.

Albers, J.J., Taggart, H.M., Applebaum-Bowden, D., Haffner, S., Chesnut, C.H., III, Hazzard, W.R. (1984). Reduction of lecithin-cholesterol acyltransferase, apolipoprotein D and the Lp(a) lipoprotein with the anabolic steroid stanozolol. *Biochimica et Biophysica Acta*, **795**, 293-296.

Alberti-Flor, C.C., Iskandarani, M., Jeffers, L., Zappa, R., & Schiff, E.R. (1984). Focal nodular hyperplasia associated with the use of a synthetic anabolic androgen. *American Journal of Gastroenterology*, **79**, 150-151.

Alen, M. (1985). Androgenic steroid effects on liver and red cells. *British Journal of Sports Medicine*, **19**, 15-20.

Alen, M., & Rahkila, P. (1984). Reduced high-density lipoprotein-cholesterol in power athletes: Use of male sex hormone derivatives, an atherogenic factor. *International Journal of Sports Medicine*, **5**, 341-342.

Alen, M., Rahkila, P., & Marniemi, J. (1985). Serum lipid in power athletes self-administering testosterone and anabolic steroids. *International Journal of Sports Medicine*, **6**, 139-144.

Alen, M., Rahkila, P., Reinila, M., & Vihko, R. (1987). Androgenic-anabolic steroid effects on serum thyroid, pituitary and steroid hormones in athletes. *American Journal of Sports Medicine*, **15**, 357-361.

American College of Sports Medicine. (1987). Position stand on the use of anabolic-androgenic steroids in sports. *Medicine and Science in Sports and Exercise*, **19**, 534-539.

Anthony, P.P. (1975). Hepatoma associated with androgenic steroids. *Lancet*, **1**, 685-686.

Appell, H.J., Heller-Umpfenbach, B., Feraudi, M., & Weicker, H. (1983). Ultrastructural and morphometric investigations on the effect of training and administration of anabolic steroids on the myocardium of guinea pigs. *International Journal of Sports Medicine, 4,* 268-274.

Applebaum, D.M., Goldberg, A.P., Pykalisto, O.J., Brunzell, J.D., & Hazzard, W.R. (1977). Effect of estrogens on postheparin plasma lipolytic activity: Selective decline in hepatic triglyceride lipase. *Journal of Clinical Investigation, 59,* 601-608.

Applebaum, D.M., Haffner, S., & Hazzard, W.R. (1987). The dyslipoproteinemia of anabolic steroid therapy: Increase in hepatic triglyceride lipase precedes the decrease in high density lipoprotein$_2$ cholesterol. *Metabolism, 36,* 949-952.

Bach, B.R., Warren, R.F., & Wickiewicz, T.L. (1987). Triceps rupture: A case report and literature review. *American Journal of Sports Medicine, 15,* 285-289.

Bagheri, S.A., & Boyer, J.L. (1974). Peliosis hepatis associated with androgenic-anabolic steroid therapy—A severe form of hepatic injury. *Annals of Internal Medicine, 81,* 610-618.

Bain, J., Rachlis, V., Robert, E., & Khait, Z. (1980). The combined use of oral medroxyprogesterone acetate and methyltestosterone in a male contraceptive trial programme. *Contraception, 21,* 365-379.

Barbosa, J., Seal, U.S., & Doe, R.P. (1971). Effects of anabolic steroids on haptoglobin, orosomucoid, plasminogen, fibrinogen, transferrin, ceruloplasmin, a1-antitrypsin, b-glucuronidase and total serum proteins. *Journal of Clinical Endocrinology, 33,* 388-398.

Bernstein, M.S., Hunter, R.L., & Yachnin, S. (1971). Hepatoma and peliosis hepatis developing in a patient with Fanconi's anemia. *New England Journal of Medicine, 284,* 1135-1136.

Bird, D., Vowles, K., & Anthony, P.P. (1979). Spontaneous rupture of a liver cell adenoma after long term methyltestosterone: Report of a case successfully treated by emergency right hepatic lobectomy. *British Journal of Surgery, 66,* 212-213.

Bonner, C.D., & Homburger, F. (1952). Jaundice of the hepatocellular type during methyltestosterone therapy: Report of two cases. *Bulletin of the New England Medical Centers, 14,* 87-89.

Burger, R.A., & Marcuse, P.M. (1952). Peliosis hepatis: Report of a case. *American Journal of Clinical Pathology, 22,* 569-573.

Burkett, L.N., & Falduto, M.T. (1984). Steroid use by athletes in a metropolitan area. *The Physician and Sportsmedicine, 12,* 69-74.

Calabrese, L.H., Kleiner, S.M., Barna, B.P., Skibinski, C.I., Kirkendall, D.T., Lahita, R.G., & Lombardo, J.A. (1989). The effects of anabolic steroids and strength training on the human immune response. *Medicine and Science in Sports and Exercise, 21,* 386-392.

Cancer of the prostate. (1954). *Journal of the American Medical Association, 156,* 292.

Carrasco, D., Prieto, M., Pallardo, L., Moll, J.L., Cruz, J.M., Munoz, C., & Berenguer, J. (1985). Multiple hepatic adenomas after long-term therapy with testosterone enanthate: Review of the literature. *Journal of Hepatology, 1,* 573-578.

Catlin, D.H., Kammerer, R.C., Hatton, C.K., Sekera, M.H., & Merdink, J.L. (1987). Analytical chemistry at the games of the XXIIIrd Olympiad in Los Angeles, 1984. *Clinical Chemistry, 33,* 319-327.

Cattan, D., Kalifat, R., Wautier, J.L., Meignan, S., Vesin, P., & Piet, R. (1974). Fanconi's anemia and primary carcinoma of the liver. *Archives Francaises des Maladies de l'Appareil Digestif, 63,* 41-48.

Cattan, D., Vesin, P., Wautier, J., Kalifat, P., & Meignan, S. (1974). Liver tumors and steroid hormones. *Lancet, 1,* 878.

Chandra, R.S., Kapur, S.P., Kelleher, J., Jr., Luban, J., & Patterson, K. (1984). Benign hepatocellular tumors in the young. A clinicopathologic spectrum. *Archives of Pathology and Laboratory Medicine, 108,* 168-171.

Charny, C.W., & Gordon, J.A. (1978). Testosterone rebound therapy: A neglected modality. *Fertility and Sterility, 29,* 64-68.

Cocks, J.R. (1981). Methyltestosterone-induced liver-cell tumours. *Medical Journal of Australia, 2,* 617-619.

Cohen, J.C., Faber, W.M., Benade, A.J., & Noakes, T.D. (1986). Altered serum lipoprotein profiles in male and female power lifters ingesting anabolic steroids. *The Physician and Sportsmedicine, 14,* 131-136.

Cohen, J.C., & Hickman, R. (1987). Insulin resistance and diminished glucose tolerance in powerlifters ingesting anabolic steroids. *Journal of Clinical Endocrinology and Metabolism, 64,* 960-963.

Cohen, J.C., Noakes, T.D., & Benade, A.J. (1988). Hypercholesteremia in male power lifters using anabolic-androgenic steroids. *The Physician and Sportsmedicine, 16,* 49-56.

Collaborative Group for the Study of Stroke in Young Women. (1975). Oral contraceptives and stroke in young women. *Journal of the American Medical Association, 231,* 718-722.

Coombes, G.B., Reiser, J., Paradinas, F., & Burn, I. (1977). An androgenic-associated hepatic adenoma in a trans-sexual. *British Journal of Surgery, 65,* 869-870.

Coronary Drug Project Research Group. (1973). The coronary drug project: Findings leading to discontinuation of the 2.5-mg/day estrogen group. *Journal of the American Medical Association, 226,* 652-657.

Costill, D.L., Pearson, D.R., & Fink, W.J. (1984). Anabolic steroid use among athletes: Changes in HDL-C levels. *The Physician and Sportsmedicine, 12,* 113-117.

Cowart, V. (1987). Steroids in sports: After four decades, time to return these genies to bottle? *Journal of the American Medical Association, 257,* 421-427.

Craig, J.R., Peters, R.L., & Edmondson, H.A. (1989). *Atlas of tumor pathology, second series, Fascicle 26: Tumors of the liver and intrahepatic bile ducts* (pp. 36-41). Washington DC: Armed Forces Institute of Pathology.

Creagh, T.M., Rubin, A., & Evans, D.J. (1988). Hepatic tumours induced by anabolic steroids in an athlete. *Journal of Clinical Pathology, 41,* 441-443.

Daneshmend, T.K., & Bradfield, J.W. (1979). Hepatic angiosarcoma associated with androgenic-anabolic steroids. *Lancet*, **2**, 1249.

Drew, E.J. (1984). Androgen related primary hepatic carcinoma in a patient on long term methyltestosterone therapy. *Journal of Abdominal Surgery*, **26**, 103-106.

Dunning, M.F. (1958). Jaundice associated with norethandrolone (Nilevar) administration. *Journal of the American Medical Association*, **167**, 1242-1243.

Edis, A.J., & Levitt, M. (1985). Anabolic steroids and colonic cancer. *Medical Journal of Australia*, **142**, 426-427.

Evely, R.S., Triger, D.R., Milnes, J.P., Low-Beer, T.S., & Williams, R. (1987). Severe cholestasis associated with stanozolol. *British Medical Journal*, **294**, 612-613.

Falk, H., Thomas, L.B., Popper, H., & Ishak, K.G. (1979). Hepatic angiosarcoma associated with androgenic-anabolic steroids. *Lancet*, **2**, 1120-1123.

Fearnley, G.R., & Chakrabarti, R. (1962). Increase of blood fibrinolytic activity by testosterone. *Lancet*, **2**, 128-132.

Fearnley, G.R., & Chakrabarti, R. (1964). The pharmacological enhancement of blood fibrinolytic activity with special reference to phenoformin. *Acta Cardiologica*, **19**, 1-13.

Foss, G.L., & Simpson, S.L. (1959). Oral methyltestosterone and jaundice. *British Medical Journal*, **1**, 259-263.

Frankle, M.A., Cicero, G.J., & Payne, J. (1984). Use of androgenic anabolic steroids by athletes. *Journal of the American Medical Association*, **252**, 482.

Frankle, M.A., Eichberg, R., & Zachariah, S.B. (1988). Anabolic androgenic steroids and a stroke in an athlete: Case report. *Archives of Physical Medicine and Rehabilitation*, **69**, 632-633.

Freed, D.L.J., Banks, A.J., Longson, D., & Burley, D.M. (1975). Anabolic steroids in athletics: Crossover double-blind trial on weightlifters. *British Medical Journal*, **2**, 471-473.

Friedl, K.E. (1987). Unpublished observations. Interview with anabolic steroid user seeking advice after purported cessation of use.

Friedl, K.E. (1990). Reappraisal of the health risks associated with the use of high doses of oral and injectable androgenic steroids. In G.C. Lin & L. Erinoff (Eds.), *Anabolic steroid abuse* (pp. 142-177). Washington DC: U.S. Government Printing Office.

Friedl, K.E., Dettori, J.R., Hannan, C.J., Patience, T.H., & Plymate, S.R. (1991). Comparison of the effects of high dose testosterone and 19-nortestosterone to a replacement dose of testosterone on strength and body composition in normal men. *Journal of Steroid Biochemistry & Molecular Biology*, **40**, 607-612.

Friedl, K.E., Hannan, C.J., Jr., Jones, R.E., & Plymate, S.R. (1990). High-density lipoprotein cholesterol is not decreased if an aromatizable androgen is administered. *Metabolism*, **39**, 69-74.

Friedl, K.E., Jones, R.E., Hannan, C.J., Jr., & Plymate, S.R. (1989). The administration of pharmacological doses of testosterone or 19-nortestosterone to normal men is not associated with increased insulin secretion or impaired glucose tolerance. *Journal of Clinical Endocrinology and Metabolism*, **68**, 971-975.

Friedl, K.E., & Plymate, S.R. (1986). Parallel profound decrease in HDL-cholesterol and testosterone binding globulin during anabolic steroid self-administration in bodybuilders. Unpublished raw data.

Friedl, K.E., & Yesalis, C.E. (1989). Self-treatment of gynecomastia in bodybuilders who use anabolic steroids. *The Physician and Sportsmedicine*, **17**, 67-79.

Furman, R.H., Howard, R.P., Norcia, L.N., & Keaty, E.C. (1958). The influence of androgens, estrogens and related steroids on serum lipids and lipoproteins: Observations in hypogonadal and normal human subjects. *American Journal of Medicine*, **24**, 80-97.

Furman, R.H., Howard, R.P., Smith, C.W., & Norcia, L.N. (1957). Comparative androgenicity of oral androgens, determined by steroid-induced decrements in high density (alpha) lipoproteins: Studies utilizing testosterone, methyltestosterone, 19-nortestosterone, 17-methyl nortestosterone and 17-ethyl nortestosterone. *American Journal of Medicine*, **22**, 966.

Garn, S.M. (1951). Types and distribution of the hair in man. *Annals of the New York Academy of Sciences*, **53**, 498-507.

Gil, V.G., Lapuerta, J.B., Garcia, J.P., & Martin, M.R. (1986). A non-C17-alkylated steroid and long-term cholestasis. *Annals of Internal Medicine*, **104**, 135-136.

Gilbert, E.F., DaSilva, A.Q., & Queen, D.M. (1963). Intrahepatic cholestasis with fatal termination following norethandrolone therapy. *Journal of the American Medical Association*, **185**, 538-539.

Gittes, R.F. (1991). Carcinoma of the prostate. *New England Journal of Medicine*, **324**, 236-245.

Glass, A.R., & Vigersky, R.A. (1980). Resensitization of testosterone production in men after human chorionic gonadotropin-induced desensitization. *Journal of Clinical Endocrinology and Metabolism*, **51**, 1395-1400.

Goldman, B. (1985). Liver carcinoma in an athlete taking anabolic steroids. *Journal of the American Osteopathic Association*, **85**, 56.

Goodman, M.A., & Laden, A.M. (1977). Hepatocellular carcinoma in association with androgen therapy. *Medical Journal of Australia*, **1**, 220-221.

Gordon, B.S., Wolf, J., Krause, T., & Shai, F. (1960). Peliosis hepatis and cholestasis following administration of norethandrolone. *American Journal of Clinical Pathology*, **33**, 156-165.

Grasso, M., Buonaguidi, A., Mondina, R., Borsellino, G., Lania, C., Banfi, G., & Rigatti, P. (1990). Plasma sex hormone binding globulin in patients with prostatic carcinoma. *Cancer*, **66**, 354-357.

Groos, G., Arnold, O.H., & Brittinger, G. (1974). Peliosis hepatis after long-term administration of oxymetholone. *Lancet*, **1**, 874.

Hamilton, J.B. (1948). The role of testicular secretions as indicated by the effects of castration in man and by studies of pathological conditions and the short lifespan associated with maleness. *Recent Progress in Hormone Research, 3*, 257-322.

Hannan, C.J., Jr., Friedl, K.E., Zold, A., Kettler, T.M., & Plymate, S.R. (1991). Psychological and serum homovanillic acid changes in men administered androgenic steroids. *Psychoneuroendocrinology, 16*, 335-343.

Haupt, H.A., & Rovere, G.D. (1984). Anabolic steroids: A review of the literature. *American Journal of Sports Medicine, 12*, 469-484.

Heller, C.G., Moore, D.J., Paulsen, C.A., Nelson, W.O., & Laidley, W.M. (1959). Progesterone and synthetic progestins: Effects of progesterone and synthetic progestins on the reproductive physiology of normal men. *Federation Proceedings, 18*, 1057-1064.

Heller, R.F., Miller, N.E., Wheeler, M.J., & Kind, P.R. (1983). Coronary heart disease in "low risk" men. *Atherosclerosis, 49*, 187-193.

Hernandez-Nieto, L., Bruguera, M., Bombi, J.A., Camacho, L., & Rozman, C. (1977). Benign liver-cell adenoma associated with long-term administration of an androgenic-anabolic steroid (methandienone). *Cancer, 40*, 1761-1764.

Hervey, G.R., Hutchinson, I., Knibbs, A.V., Burkinshaw, L., Jones, P.R., Nolan, N.G., & Levell, M.J. (1976). "Anabolic" effects of methandienone in men undergoing athletic training. *Lancet, 2*, 699-702.

Hill, J.A., Suker, J.R., Sachs, K., & Brigham, C. (1983). The athletic polydrug abuse phenomenon. *American Journal of Sports Medicine, 11*, 269-271.

Hobbs, C.J., Plymate, S.R., Bell, B.K., & Patience, T.H. (1991). The effect of androgens on glucose tolerance. *Clinical Research, 39*, 384A.

Hobbs, C.J., Plymate, S.R., Jones, R.E., Andress, D.L., & Patience, T.H. (1991). The effect of androgens on insulin-like growth factor-I levels in normal men. *Clinical Research, 39*, 55A.

Hurley, B.F., Seals, D.R., Hagberg, J.M., Goldberg, A.C., Ostrove, S.M., Holloszy, J.O., Wiest, W.G., & Goldberg, A.P. (1984). High-density-lipoprotein cholesterol in bodybuilders v. powerlifters: Negative effects of androgen use. *Journal of the American Medical Association, 252*, 507-513.

Ingerowski, G.H., Scheutwinkel-Reich, M., & Stan, H.J. (1981). Mutagenicity studies on veterinary anabolic drugs with the salmonella/microsome test. *Mutation Research, 91*, 93-98.

Jarow, J.P., & Lipshultz, L.I. (1990). Anabolic steroid-induced hypogonadotropic hypogonadism. *American Journal of Sports Medicine, 18*, 429-431.

Johnsen, S.G., Bennett, E.P., & Jensen, V.G. (1974). Therapeutic effectiveness of oral testosterone. *Lancet, 2*, 1473-1475.

Johnsen, S.G., Kampmann, J.P., Bennett, E.P., & Jorgensen, F.S. (1976). Enzyme induction by oral testosterone. *Clinical Pharmacology and Therapeutics, 20*, 233-237.

Johnson, F.L., Lerner, K.G., Siegel, M., Faegler, J.R., Majerus, P.W., Hartmann, J.R., & Thomas, E.D. (1972). Association of androgenic-anabolic steroid therapy with development of hepatocellular carcinoma. *Lancet*, **2**, 1273-1276.

Joint Group for the Study of Aplastic and Refractory Anemias. (1981). Long-term follow-up of patients with medullary aplasia. *Annales de Medicine Interne*, **132**, 530-534.

Jurgens, G., & Koltringer, P. (1987). Lipoprotein(a) in ischemic cerebrovascular disease: A new approach to the assessment of risk for stroke. *Neurology*, **37**, 513-515.

Kantor, M.A., Bianchini, A., Bernier, D., Sady, S.P., & Thompson, P.D. (1985). Androgens reduce HDL2-cholesterol and increase hepatic triglyceride lipase activity. *Medicine and Science in Sports and Exercise*, **17**, 462-465.

Karasawa, T., Shikata, T., & Smith, R.D. (1979). Peliosis hepatis: Report of nine cases. *Acta Pathologica Japonica*, **29**, 457-469.

Kessler, E., Bar-Meir, S., & Pinkhas, J. (1976). Focal nodular hyperplasia and spontaneous hepatic rupture in aplastic anemia treated with oxymetholone. *Harefuah*, **90**, 521-524.

Kintzen, W., & Silny, J. (1960). Peilosis hepatis after administration of fluoxymesterone. *Canadian Medical Association Journal*, **83**, 860-862.

Kiraly, C.L. (1988). Androgenic-anabolic steroid effects on serum and skin surface lipids, on red cells, and on liver enzymes. *International Journal of Sports Medicine*, **9**, 249-252.

Kiraly, C.L., Alen, M., Rahkila, P., & Horsmanheimo, M. (1987). Effect of androgenic and anabolic steroids on the sebaceous gland in power athletes. *Acta Dermatologica et Venereologica*, **67**, 36-40.

Klatskin, G. (1977). Hepatic tumors: Possible relationship to use of oral contraceptives. *Gastroenterology*, **73**, 386-394.

Kloer, H., Hoogen, H., & Nieschlag, E. (1980). Trial of high-dose testosterone undecanoate in treatment of male infertility. *International Journal of Andrology*, **3**, 121-129.

Knuth, U.A., Maniera, H., & Nieschlag, E. (1989). Anabolic steroids and semen parameters in bodybuilders. *Acta Endocrinologica*, **120**(Suppl.), 121-122.

Kory, R.C., Bradley, M.H., Watson, R.N., Callahan, R., & Peters, B.J. (1959). A six-month evaluation of an anabolic drug, norethandrolone, in underweight persons: 2. Brosulphalein (BSP) retention and liver function. *American Journal of Medicine*, **26**, 243-248.

Koszalka, M.F. (1957). Medical obstructive jaundice: Report of death due to methyltestosterone. *Lancet*, **77**, 51-54.

Kramhoft, M., & Solgaard, S. (1986). Spontaneous rupture of the extensor pollicis longus tendon after anabolic steroids. *Journal of Hand Surgery*, **11**, 87.

Kruskemper, H.L. (1968). *Anabolic steroids* (p. 176). New York: Academic Press.

Landon, J., Wynn, V., Cooke, J.N., & Kennedy, A. (1962). Effects of anabolic steroid methandienone, on carbohydrate metabolism in man. *Metabolism*, **11**, 501-512.

Landon, J., Wynn, V., & Samols, E. (1963). The effect of anabolic steroids on blood sugar and plasma insulin levels in man. *Metabolism*, **12**, 924-935.

Laroche, G.P. (1990). Steroid anabolic drugs and arterial complications in an athlete—a case history. *Angiology*, **41**, 964-969.

Lenders, J.W., Demacker, P.N., Vos, J.A., Jansen, P.L., Hoitsma, A.J., van't Laar, A., & Thien, T. (1988). Deleterious effects of anabolic steroids on serum lipoproteins, blood pressure, and liver function in amateur body builders. *International Journal of Sports Medicine*, **9**, 19-23.

Lesna, M., & Taylor, W. (1986). Liver lesions in BALB/C mice induced by an anabolic androgen (Decadurabolin), with and without pretreatment with diethylnitrosamine. *Journal of Steroid Biochemistry*, **24**, 449-453.

Lichtenstein, M.J., Yarnell, J.W., Elwood, P.C., Beswick, A.D., Sweetnam, P.M., Marks, V., Teale, D., & Riad-Fahmy, D. (1987). Sex hormones, insulin, lipids, and prevalent ischemic heart disease. *American Journal of Epidemiology*, **126**, 647-657.

Liddle, G.W., & Burke, H.A. (1960). Anabolic steroids in clinical medicine. *Helvetica Medica Acta*, **27**, 504-513.

Lloyd-Thomas, H.G., & Sherlock, S. (1952). Testosterone therapy for the pruritis of obstructive jaundice. *British Medical Journal*, **2**, 1289.

Loomus, G.N., Aneja, P., & Bota, R.A. (1983). A case of peliosis hepatis in association with tamoxifen therapy. *American Journal of Clinical Pathology*, **80**, 881-883.

Lowdell, C.P., & Murray-Lyon, I.M. (1985). Reversal of liver damage due to long term methyltestosterone and safety of non-17a-alkylated androgens. *British Medical Journal*, **291**, 637.

Luke, J.L., Farb, A., Virmani, R., & Sample, R.H. (1990). Sudden cardiac death during exercise in a weight lifter using anabolic androgenic steroids: Pathological and toxicology findings. *Journal of Forensic Sciences*, **35**, 1441-1447.

Martikainen, H., Alen, M., Rahkila, P., & Vihko, R. (1986). Testicular responsiveness to human chorionic gonadotrophin during transient hypogonadotrophic hypogonadism induced by androgenic/anabolic steroids in power athletes. *Journal of Steroid Biochemistry*, **25**, 109-112.

Matsumoto, A.M. (1988). Is high dosage testosterone an effective male contraceptive agent? *Fertility and Sterility*, **50**, 324-328.

Matsumoto, A.M. (1990). Effects of chronic testosterone administration in normal men: Safety and efficacy of high dosage testosterone and parallel dose-dependent suppression of luteinizing hormone, follicle-stimulating hormone, and sperm production. *Journal of Clinical Endocrinology and Metabolism*, **70**, 282-287.

Matsumoto, A.M., & Bremner, W.J. (1988). Parallel dose-dependent suppression of LH, FSH and sperm production by testosterone in normal men. Abstract No. 570, p. 163, Proceedings of the 70th Annual Meeting of the Endocrine Society, The Endocrine Society, Bethesda, MD.

Mauss, J., Borsch, G., Bormacher, K., Richter, E., Leyendecker, G., & Nocke, W. (1975). Effect of long-term testosterone enanthate administration on male reproduction function: Clinical evaluation, serum FSH, LH, testosterone, and seminal fluid analyses in normal men. *Acta Endocrinologica*, **78**, 373-384.

McCaughan, G.W., Bilous, M.J., & Gallagher, N.D. (1985). Long-term survival with tumor regression in androgen-induced liver tumors. *Cancer*, **56**, 2622-2626.

McKillop, G., Todd, I.C., & Ballantyne, D. (1986). Increased left ventricular mass in a bodybuilder using anabolic steroids. *British Journal of Sports Medicine*, **20**, 151-152.

McNutt, R.A., Ferenchick, G.S., Kirlin, P.C., & Hamlin, N.J. (1988). Acute myocardial infarction in a 22-year-old world class weight lifter using anabolic steroids. *American Journal of Cardiology*, **62**, 164.

Messerli, F.H., & Frohlich, E.D. (1979). High blood pressure: A side effect of drugs, poisons, and food. *Archives of Internal Medicine*, **139**, 682-687.

Michna, H. (1987). Tendon injuries induced by exercise and anabolic steroids in experimental mice. *International Orthopaedics*, **11**, 157-162.

Mochizuki, R.M., & Richter, K.J. (1988). Cardiomyopathy and cerebrovascular accident associated with anabolic-androgenic steroid use. *The Physician and Sportsmedicine*, **16**, 109-114.

Nadell, J., & Kosek, J. (1977). Peliosis hepatis. Twelve cases associated with oral androgen therapy. *Archives of Pathology and Laboratory Medicine*, **101**, 405-410.

Nagelberg, S.B., Laue, L., Loriaux, D.L., Liu, L., & Sherins, R.J. (1986). Cerebrovascular accident associated with testosterone therapy in a 21-year-old hypogonadal man. *New England Journal of Medicine*, **314**, 649-650.

National Cholesterol Education Program Expert Panel. (1988). Report of the National Cholesterol Education Program Expert Panel on detection, evaluation, and treatment of high blood cholesterol in adults. *Archives of Internal Medicine*, **148**, 36-69.

Neff, M.S., Goldberg, J., Slifkin, R.F., Eiser, A.R., Calamia, V., Kaplan, M., Baez, A., Gupta, S., & Mattoo, N. (1981). A comparison of androgens for anemia in patients on hemodialysis. *New England Journal of Medicine*, **304**, 871-875.

Nelson, W.O. (1959). Progesterone and synthetic progestins: Discussion. *Federation Proceedings*, **18**, 1065.

Noble, R.L. (1984). Androgen use by athletes: A possible cancer risk. *Canadian Medical Association Journal*, **130**, 549-550.

Overly, W.L., Dankoff, J.A., Wang, B.K., & Singh, U.D. (1984). Androgens and hepatocellular carcinoma in an athlete. *Annals of Internal Medicine*, **100**, 158-159.

Palacios, A., McClure, R.D., Campfield, A., & Swerdloff, R.S. (1981). Effect of testosterone enanthate on testis size. *Journal of Urology*, **126**, 46-48.

Paradinas, F.J., Bull, T.B., Westaby, D., & Murray-Lyon, I.M. (1977). Hyperplasia and prolapse of hepatocytes into hepatic veins during long term methyltestosterone therapy: Possible relationships of these changes to the development of peliosis hepatis and liver tumors. *Histopathology*, **1**, 225-226.

Paulsen, C.A., Bremner, W.J., & Leonard, J.M. (1982). Male contraception: Clinical trials. In D.R. Mishell (Ed.), *Advances in fertility research* (pp. 157-170). New York: Raven Press.

Pecking, A., Lejolly, J.M., & Najean, Y. (1980). Hepatic toxicity of androgen therapy in aplastic anemia. *Nouvelle Revue Francaise d'Hematologie*, **22**, 257-265.

Pelletier, G., Frija, J., Szekely, A.M., & Clauvel, J.P. (1984). Adenoma of the liver in man. *Gastroenterologie Clinique et Biologique*, **8**, 269-272.

Pelliccia, A., Maron, B.J., Spataro, A., Proschan, M.A., & Spirito, P. (1991). The upper limit of physiologic cardiac hypertrophy in highly trained elite athletes. *New England Journal of Medicine*, **324**, 295-301.

Petera, V., Bobek, K., & Lahn, V. (1962). Serum transaminase (GOT,GPT) and lactic dehydrogenase activity during treatment with methyl testosterone. *Clinica Chimica Acta*, **7**, 604-606.

Peters, J.H., Randall, A.H., Mendeloff, J., Peace, R., Coberly, J.C., & Hurley, M.B. (1958). Jaundice during administration of methylestrenolone. *Journal of Clinical Endocrinology and Metabolism*, **18**, 114-115.

Peters, R.L. (1976). Pathology of hepatocellular carcinoma. In K. Okuda & R.L. Peters (Eds.), *Hepatocellular carcinoma* (pp. 107-168). New York: Wiley.

Peterson, G.E., & Fahey, T.D. (1984). HDL-C in five elite athletes using anabolic-androgenic steroids. *The Physician and Sportsmedicine*, **12**, 120-130.

Petry, R., Rausch-Stroomann, J.G., Hienz, H.A., Senge, T., & Mauss, J. (1968). Androgen treatment without inhibiting effect on hypophysis and male gonads. *Acta Endocrinologica*, **59**, 497-507.

Phillips, M.J., Oda, M., & Funatsu, K. (1978). Evidence for microfilament involvement in norethandrolone-induced intrahepatic cholestasis. *American Journal of Pathology*, **93**, 729-744.

Pochi, P.E., Strauss, J.S. (1974). Endocrinologic control of the development and activity of the human sebaceous gland. *Journal of Investigative Dermatology*, **62**, 191-201.

Prat, J., Gray, G.F., Stolley, P.D., & Coleman, J.W. (1977). Wilms tumor in an adult associated with androgen abuse. *Journal of the American Medical Association*, **237**, 2322-2323.

Rastad, J., Joborn, H., Ljunghall, S., & Akerstrom, G. (1985). Gluteal infection in weight lifters after injection of anabolic steroids. *Lakartidningen*, **82**, 3407. (DIALOG b 155 8639139)

Roberts, J.T., & Essenhigh, D.M. (1986). Adenocarcinoma of prostate in 40-year-old body-builder. *Lancet*, **2**, 742.

Ross, R., Bernstein, L., Judd, H., Hanisch, R., Pike, M., & Henderson, B. (1986). Serum testosterone levels in healthy young black and white men. *Journal of the National Cancer Institute*, **76**, 45-48.

Rowley, M.J., & Heller, C.G. (1972). The testosterone rebound phenomenon in the treatment of male infertility. *Fertility and Sterility*, **23**, 498-504.

Rozenek, R., Rahe, C.H., Kohl, H.H., Marple, D.N., Wilson, G.D., & Stone, M.H. (1990). Physiological responses to resistance-exercise in athletes self-administering anabolic steroids. *The Journal of Sports Medicine and Physical Fitness*, **30**, 354-360.

Ruokonen, A., Alen, M., Bolton, N., & Vihko, R. (1985). Response of serum testosterone and its precursor steroids, SHBG and CBG to anabolic steroid and testosterone self-administration in man. *Journal of Steroid Biochemistry*, **23**, 33-38.

Saartok, T., Dahlberg, E., & Gustafsson, J.A. (1984). Relative binding affinity of anabolic-androgenic steroids: Comparison of the binding to the androgen receptors in skeletal muscle and in prostate, as well as to sex hormone-binding globulin. *Endocrinology*, **114**, 2100-2106.

Saheb, F. (1980). Absence of peliosis hepatis in patients receiving testosterone enanthate. *Hepato-Gastroenterology*, **27**, 432-434.

Sale, G.E., & Lerner, K.G. (1977). Multiple tumors after androgen therapy. *Archives of Pathology and Laboratory Medicine*, **101**, 600-603.

Salke, R.C., Rowland, T.W., & Burke, E.J. (1985). Left ventricular size and function in body builders using anabolic steroids. *Medicine and Science in Sports and Exercise*, **17**, 701-704.

Schaffner, F., Popper, H., & Chesrow, E. (1959). Cholestasis produced by the administration of norethandrolone. *American Journal of Medicine*, **26**, 249-254.

Schaison, G., Leverger, G., & Yildez, C. (1983). Fanconi's anemia: Frequency of leukemic transformation. *Presse Medicin*, **12**, 1269-1274.

Schally, A.V., & Comaru-Schally, A.M. (1987). Male contraception involving testosterone supplementation: Possible increased risks of prostate cancer? *Lancet*, **1**, 448-449.

Schriewer, H., Assmann, G., Sandkamp, M., & Schulte, H. (1984). The relationship of lipoprotein(a) (Lp(a)) to risk factors of coronary heart disease: Initial results of the prospective epidemiological study on company employees in Westfalia. *Journal of Clinical Chemistry and Clinical Biochemistry*, **22**, 591-596.

Schurmeyer, T., Knuth, U.A., Belkien, L., Nieschlag, E. (1984). Reversible azzospermia induced by the anabolic steroid 19-nortestosterone. *Lancet*, **1**, 417-420.

Scott, M.J., & Scott, M.J., Jr. (1989). HIV infection associated with injections of anabolic steroids. *Journal of the American Medical Association*, **262**, 207-298.

Scully, R.E., Mark, E.J., & McNeely, B.U. (1981). Weekly clinico-pathological exercises: Case 32-1981. *New England Journal of Medicine, 305,* 331-336.

Schiozawa, Z., Tsunoda, S., Noda, A., Saito, M., & Yamada, H. (1986). Cerebral hemorrhagic infarction associated with anabolic steroid therapy for hypoplastic anemia. *Angiology, 37,* 725-730.

Shiozawa, Z., Yamada, H., Mabuchi, C., Hotta, T., Saito, M., Sobue, I., & Huang, Y.P. (1982). Superior sagittal sinus thrombosis associated with androgen therapy for hypoplastic anemia. *Annals of Neurology, 12,* 578-580.

Simon, M., Jouet, J.P., Demory, J.L., Pollet, J.P., & Bauters, F. (1986). An unrecognized cause of polycythemia: Prolonged anabolic drug treatment. *Presse Medicale, 15,* 396.

Sklarek, H.M., Mantovani, R.P., Erens, E., Heisler, D., Niederman, M.S., & Fein, A.M. (1984). AIDS in a bodybuilder using anabolic steroids. *New England Journal of Medicine, 311,* 1701.

Spano, F., & Ryan, W.G. (1984). Tamoxifen for gynecomastia induced by anabolic steroids? *New England Journal of Medicine, 311,* 861-862.

Stalder, M., Pometta, D., & Suenram, A. (1981). Relationship between plasma insulin levels and high density lipoprotein cholesterol levels in healthy men. *Diabetologia, 21,* 544-548.

Steinberger, E., Smith, K.D., & Rodriguez-Rigau, L.J. (1978). Suppression and recovery of sperm production in men treated with testosterone enanthate for one year. A study of a possible reversible male contraceptive. *International Journal of Andrology, 2*(Suppl.), 748-760.

Strauss, J.S., & Pochi, P.E. (1963). III. Hormones and cellular metabolism: The human sebaceous gland: Its regulation by steroidal hormones and its use as an end organ for assaying androgenicity in vivo. *Recent Progress in Hormone Research, 19,* 385-444.

Strauss, R.H., Wright, J.E., Finerman, G.A., & Catlin, D.H. (1983). Side effects of anabolic steroids in weight-trained men. *The Physician and Sportsmedicine, 11,* 87-96.

Svanborg, A., & Ohlsson, S. (1959). Recurrent jaundice of pregnancy: A clinical study of twenty-two cases. *American Journal of Medicine, 27,* 40-49.

Sweeney, E.C., & Evans, D.J. (1976). Hepatic lesions in patients treated with synthetic anabolic steroids. *Journal of Clinical Pathology, 29,* 623-626.

Swerdloff, R.S., Palacios, A., McClure, R.D., Campfield, L.A., & Brosman, S.A. (1978). Male contraception: Clinical assessment of chronic administration of testosterone enanthate. *International Journal of Andrology, 2*(Suppl.), 731-747.

Taxy, J.B. (1978). Peliosis: A morphologic curiosity becomes an iatrogenic problem. *Human Pathology, 9,* 331-340.

Thompson, P.D., Culinane, E.M., Sady, S.P., Chenevert, C., Saritelli, A.L., Sady, M.A., & Herbert, P.N. (1989). Contrasting effects of testosterone and stanozolol on serum lipoprotein levels. *Journal of the American Medical Association*, **261**, 1165-1168.

Tikkanen, M.J., Nikkila, E.A., Kussi, T., & Sipinen, S. (1982). High density lipoprotein-2 and hepatic lipase: Reciprocal changes produced by estrogen and norgestrel. *Journal of Clinical Endocrinology and Metabolism*, **54**, 1113-1117.

Treuner, J., Niethammer, D., Flach, A., Fischbach, H., & Schenck, W. (1980). Hepatocellular carcinoma after oxymetholone treatment. *Medizinische Welt*, **31**, 952-955.

Turani, H., Levi, J., Zevin, D., & Kessler, E. (1983). Hepatic lesions in patients on anabolic androgenic therapy. *Israel Journal of Medical Sciences*, **19**, 332-337.

Verwilghen, R., Louwagie, A., Waes, J., & Vandenbroucke, J. (1966). Anabolic agents and relative polycythemia. *British Journal of Haematology*, **12**, 712-716.

Vesselinovitch, S.D., & Mihailovich, N. (1967). The effect of gonadectomy on the development of hepatomas induced by urethane. *Cancer Research*, **27**, 1788-1791.

Vessey, M., Doll, R., Peto, R., Johnson, B., & Wiggins, P. (1976). A long-term follow-up study of women using different methods of contraception—an interim report. *Journal of Biosocial Science*, **8**, 373-427.

Wakabayashi, T., Onda, H., Tada, T., Iijima, M., & Itoh, Y. (1984). High incidence of peliosis hepatis in autopsy cases of aplastic anemia with special reference to anabolic steroid therapy. *Acta Pathologica Japonica*, **34**, 1079-1086.

Webb, O.L., Laskarzewski, P.M., & Glueck, C.J. (1984). Severe depression of high-density lipoprotein cholesterol levels in weight lifters and body builders by self-administered exogenous testosterone and anabolic-androgenic steroids. *Metabolism*, **33**, 971-975.

Weider, J. (1987). How drugs affect peaking. *Muscle & Fitness*, **49**, 150-153, 232-233.

Weinbauer, G.F., Marshall, G.R., & Nieschlag, E. (1986). New injectable testosterone ester maintains serum testosterone of castrated monkeys in the normal range for four months. *Acta Endocrinologica*, **113**, 128-132.

Werner, S.C. (1947). Clinical syndromes associated with gonadal failure in men. *American Journal of Medicine*, **3**, 52-66.

Werner, S.C., Hanger, F.M., & Kritzler, R. (1950). Jaundice during methyl testosterone therapy. *American Journal of Medicine*, **8**, 325-331.

Westaby, D., Ogle, S.J., Paradinas, F.J., Randell, J.B., & Murray-Lyon, I.M. (1977). Liver damage from long-term methyltestosterone. *Lancet*, **1**, 261-263.

Westaby, D., Portmann, B., & Williams, R. (1983). Androgen related primary hepatic tumors in non-Fanconi patients. *Cancer*, **51**, 1947-1952.

Wilson, J.D., Aiman, J., & MacDonald, P.C. (1980). Pathogenesis of gynecomastia. *Advances in Internal Medicine*, **25**, 1-32.

Wing, T.Y., Ewing, L.L., Zegeye, B., & Zirkin, B.R. (1985). Restoration effects of exogenous luteinizing hormone on the testicular steroidogenesis and Leydig cell ultrastructure. *Endocrinology*, **117**, 1779-1787.

Winwood, P.J., Robertson, D.A.F., Wright, R. (1990). Bleeding oesophageal varices associated with anabolic steroid use in an athlete. *Postgraduate Medicine*, **66**, 864-865.

Woodard, T.L., Burghen, G.A., Kitabchi, A.E., & Wilimas, J.A. (1981). Glucose intolerance and insulin resistance in aplastic anemia treated with oxymetholone. *Journal of Clinical Endocrinology and Metabolism*, **53**, 905-908.

World Health Organization Task Force on Methods for the Regulation of Male Fertility. (1990). Contraceptive efficacy of testosterone-induced azoospermia in normal men. *Lancet*, **336**, 955-959.

Wynn, V., Landon, J., & Kawerau, E. (1961). Studies on hepatic function during methandienone therapy. *Lancet*, **1**, 69-75.

Yesalis, C.E., Herrick, R.T., Buckley, W.E., Friedl, K.E., Brannon, D., & Wright, J.E. (1988). Self-reported use of anabolic-androgenic steroids by elite power lifters. *The Physician and Sportsmedicine*, **16**, 91-100.

Zuliani, U., Bernardini, B., Catapano, A., Campana, M., Cerioli, G., & Spattini, G. (1989). Effects of anabolic steroids, testosterone, and HGH on blood lipids and echocardiographic parameters in body builders. *International Journal of Sports Medicine*, **10**, 62-66.

CHAPTER 7

Additional Effects of Anabolic Steroids on Women

Richard H. Strauss
Charles E. Yesalis

All synthetic anabolic steroids are able to produce virilization phenomena in women.

H.L. KRUSKEMPER
Anabolic Steroids, 1968

Anabolic steroids, also known as anabolic-androgenic steroid hormones or simply as androgens (see chapter 1), are hormones whose major effect is masculinization. The principal masculinizing hormone that occurs naturally in men—and to a lesser extent in women—is testosterone. In fact, many of the differences between men and women are due to the higher levels of testosterone in males during development or maturity (Bardin & Catteral, 1981). Estrogens secreted by the ovaries have a major effect on fat distribution, the reproductive tract, and the pelvis. But differing amounts of testosterone account for the sexual dimorphism of nonreproductive tissues in men and women.

Only a few studies have been performed on women who take androgens because relatively few women take these drugs for therapeutic or other reasons. Thus, some of our information comes from studies of disease states in which the women themselves produce excess androgens. Also, androgens occasionally have been administered as treatment for diseases in women or, in higher doses, to masculinize female-to-male transsexuals. We also note health effects of androgens on males and surmise that similar risks may apply to females who take large amounts of androgens.

In males, testosterone is produced mainly by the testes. Its production rises dramatically at puberty and results in sexual maturity, including enlargement of the penis. Increased androgen levels, particularly testosterone levels, also result in beard growth, deepening of the voice, and coarsening of the skin. Muscle size and strength are also promoted by the presence of increased levels of testosterone (Kochakian, 1976; Kruskemper, 1968). In adulthood, differences between a eunuchoid male and a normal man are the result of the latter's normally high levels of circulating androgenic hormones.

Women naturally have small amounts of circulating testosterone (Table 7.1). Other androgens, including dehydroepiandrosterone sulfate, are present in women in small amounts. These hormones are secreted primarily by the adrenal glands, although the ovaries also secrete a small amount of androgens. In human females, increased levels of testosterone are known to have masculinizing effects. For example, in the syndrome of adrenal androgen excess, elevated androgen secretion can result in a masculinized female before, during, or after puberty (Kochakian, 1976).

Androgenic hormones occasionally have been used therapeutically in women, usually in small doses. For example, danacrin has been used to treat endometriosis, and several anabolic steroids have been employed as antitumor agents in metastatic breast cancer (Kochakian, 1976). Side effects of anabolic steroid therapy in women may include deepening of the voice, facial hair growth, extension of pubic hair, hypertrophy of the clitoris, and loss of scalp hair (Kruskemper, 1968).

Table 7.1   Testosterone Plasma Levels and Production Rates in Men and Women

Category	Women	Men
Plasma levels	38-40 ng/dl	700 ng/dl
Production rates	0.3 mg/day	7 mg/day

Note. Adapted from Yen and Jaffee (1978).

In sports, men were apparently the first to use anabolic steroids in an attempt to increase strength and muscle size (see chapter 2). However, women were not far behind. Initially, women sought to increase strength and performance in events such as the shot put; subsequently, women bodybuilders wanted larger muscles (Dayton, 1990).

Patterns of Use

The use of anabolic steroids by adolescent girls in the United States appears to be low but significant. Studies at local, state, and national levels found that approximately 1% of female high school seniors had used anabolic steroids—some as early as the 6th grade (see chapter 3).

In surveys of female intercollegiate athletes, two studies (Anderson & McKeag, 1985; Anderson, Albrecht, McKeag, Hough, & McGrew, 1991) found that 1% of participants in swimming, basketball, and track and field reported using steroids in the past 12 months. When Yesalis et al. (1990) asked female intercollegiate athletes to estimate the level of steroid use among competitors in their own sports, a somewhat different picture emerged. The respondents judged that 5% of swimmers, 6% of basketball players, and 10% of track-and-field athletes had used anabolic steroids in the past 12 months. In addition, at least one-quarter of the study participants in softball, tennis, gymnastics, field hockey, volleyball, and lacrosse believed that there was some steroid use in their respective sports in the previous 12 months.

The prevalence of anabolic steroid use is thought to be high among women engaged in bodybuilding, power lifting, shot put, and other sports that depend on maximal strength. In competitions in which drug testing has been performed, women have been detected using anabolic steroids in power lifting, bodybuilding, the shot put, the javelin throw, swimming, and running (Wadler & Hainline, 1989).

Newman (1987) surveyed elite female athletes, including those competing at the Olympic, collegiate, and professional levels in more than 15 sports. The incidence of lifetime anabolic steroids use was 3%, but only 1% of subjects acknowledged using these drugs in the preceding year. The lifetime use rates were slightly higher for those women over the age of 25 (4%) and members of professional teams (5%).

In studies of female bodybuilders conducted in Sweden (Lindstrom, Nilsson, Katzman, Janzon, & Dymling, 1990) and the United States (Tricker, O'Neill, & Cook, 1989), approximately 10% acknowledged prior use of anabolic steroids. In the U.S. study, the female bodybuilders who used steroids were younger than the male users (22 years vs. 27 years), whereas the Swedish study did not report the ages of the participants.

The levels of anabolic steroid use reported by women could be underestimates due to poor communication between the athletes and the scientists, the sanctions against drug use, or disapproval of drug use by family, friends, or fans. The virilizing effects of the drugs, and how virilization is viewed by society, also may make female athletes hesitant to disclose their steroid use.

A major question is, Do anabolic steroids help women build bigger, stronger muscles? The answer is almost certainly *yes*, even though no controlled studies have tested the strength of women before and after the use of anabolic steroids. This conclusion is based on the significant effects of androgen administration on muscle in female and castrated male animals (Kochakian, 1976; Kruskemper, 1968); it is also based on the physical appearance of females with adrenogenital syndrome, discussed earlier, as well as the changes in phenotype of transsexuals administered androgens.

Muscle size may decrease when steroids are stopped, although not necessarily to the pre-use level. Of course, muscle size can diminish dramatically when physical training is stopped or with disuse and inactivity.

Drugs Used

The anabolic steroids used by 10 weight-trained women athletes (Strauss, Liggett, & Lanese, 1985) are listed in Table 7.2. Oral preparations included methandrostenolone (Dianabol) and stanozolol (Winstrol). Injectable drugs included two veterinary preparations, stanozolol (Winstrol-V) and boldenone (Equipoise). The doses ranged from a moderate amount of a single drug to the use, in one woman, of five different anabolic steroids stacked during a 10-week cycle (this is comparable to moderately heavy use in the male population [Duchaine, 1989]) (Table 7.3).

Side Effects of Anabolic Steroids

Many of the side effects noted by women are a result of the masculinizing effects of these hormones. Table 7.4 lists the side effects noted by the same 10 users whose data are shown in Tables 7.2 and 7.3. Effects included

Table 7.2   Anabolic Steroids Used in Training or Competition (10 Women)

Oral
  Mesterolone (Proviron)
  Methandrostenolone (Dianabol)
  Methenolone acetate (Primobolan)
  Methyltestosterone
  Oxandrolone (Anavar)
  Stanozolol (Winstrol)

Injectable
  Boldenone undecylenate (Equipoise; veterinary)
  Methandrostenolone ("injectable Dianabol")
  Methenolone enanthate (Primobolan)
  Nandrolone decanoate (Deca-Durabolin)
  Stanozolol (Winstrol-V; veterinary)
  Stenbolone acetate (Anatrofin)
  Testosterone cypionate
  Mixture of testosterone esters (Sustanon 250)

Note. Adapted from Strauss, Liggett, and Lanese (1985) by permission.

Table 7.3   Anabolic Steroids Reported by Heaviest User (10-Week Cycle)

Drug	Dose	Duration of use (weeks)
Oral		
Stanozolol (Winstrol)	12 mg/day	10
Oxandrolone (Anavar)	10 mg/day	10
Mesterolone (Proviron)	50 mg/day	10
Injectable		
Stanozolol (Winstrol-V, veterinary)	50 mg/2 days	last 6
Methenolone enanthate (Primobolan)	30 mg/2 days	last 4

Note. Adapted from Strauss, Liggett, and Lanese (1985) by permission.

deepening of the voice, growth of facial hair, increased body hair, and enlargement of the clitoris. These effects generally appear to be permanent and have been reported by other women bodybuilders using anabolic steroids (Tricker et al., 1989). Effects that seemed to return to normal after the androgenic hormones were stopped included menstrual cessation or irregularity, increased libido, increased aggressiveness, and acne.

Of 26 female-to-male transsexuals who received long-term androgen treatment, 69% were found to have polycystic ovaries (Spinder et al.,

Table 7.4   Perceived Side Effects of Anabolic Steroids (10 Women)

Effect	Number reporting effect
Lowered voice	10
Increased facial hair	9
Enlarged clitoris	8
Increased aggressiveness	8
Increased appetite	8
Decreased body fat	8
Diminished or stopped menstruation	7
Increased libido	6
Increased acne	6
Decreased breast size	5
Increased body hair	5
Increased loss of scalp hair	2

Note. Adapted from Strauss, Liggett, and Lanese (1985) by permission.

1989). Some women feel that menopause may be reached sooner when there is a long history of anabolic steroid use. As with men, variability exists in women's responses to anabolic steroids (Kruskemper, 1968).

Endocrine changes have been documented. In a study of nine women weight lifters who used androgens (Malarkey, Strauss, Leizmen, Liggett, & Demers, 1991), seven women injected testosterone esters, resulting in circulating levels of testosterone up to 34 times the normal female level (Figure 7.1). Three of these seven women exceeded the upper limits of normal levels for men. The nine users of oral and injectable anabolic steroids had significantly lower levels of SHBG (Figure 7.2), thyroid-binding globulins, and HDLC as compared to controls.

The health risks that are discussed in chapter 6 apply to women as well as men. In particular, the 17-alkyl-substituted androgens are associated with liver abnormalities including (rarely) tumors. Adverse changes in lipid profiles, including decreased HDLC (Malarkey et al., 1991; Moffatt, Wallace, & Sady, 1990), suggest that women users may have an increased risk for cardiovascular disease.

If a woman was pregnant with a female fetus at the time she was taking anabolic steroids, it is likely that the fetus would be masculinized, although no cases of this have been reported.

Why Do Women Use Anabolic Steroids?

In the Strauss et al. (1985) study, the researchers attempted to analyze this question by discussing it with the subjects. All 10 women reported a significant increase in muscle strength, muscle size, and sport performance

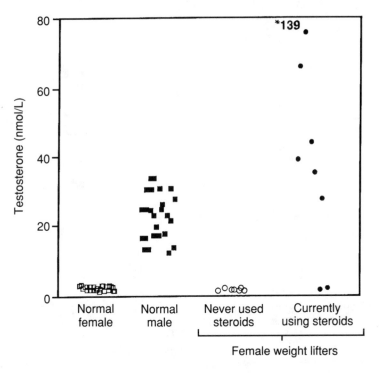

Figure 7.1 Serum testosterone levels were elevated in the seven women weight lifters who were injecting testosterone and were normal in the two women who were using only other anabolic steroids. Note that several testosterone levels in the women users were higher than those found in normal males. *Note.* Reprinted from Malarkey, Strauss, Leizmen, Liggett, and Demers (1991) by permission.

when they first began using steroids. These were the effects that the women sought, and these effects represented the participants' perceptions rather than objective measurements. The athletes continued to use steroids in a cyclical manner because they considered their sport performances to be better when they were taking steroids than when they were not.

Other perceived effects of anabolic steroids, including adverse effects, are shown in Table 7.4. Every athlete noticed that her voice became lower, and 7 of the 10 participants felt that this was undesirable. Nine of the 10 women observed increased facial hair, and all except one thought that this was undesirable. Eight participants noted clitoral enlargement, with no consensus as to the desirability of this change. Six noted increased libido, which most thought desirable. Breast size was believed to decrease in five subjects, four of whom attached no significance to this, and one who thought the decrease was desirable. Menstrual diminution or cessation was common, and there was no agreement as to the desirability of

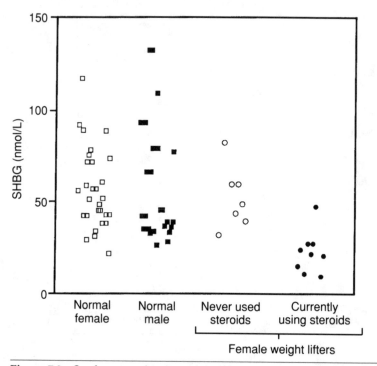

Figure 7.2   Sex hormone binding globulin levels were significantly decreased (p less than 0.02) in the women who were using anabolic steroids. *Note.* Reprinted from Malarkey, Strauss, Leizmen, Liggett, and Demers (1991) by permission.

this. Eight women noted increased aggressiveness, six of whom felt this was desirable because it enhanced their drive to practice and compete. However, some reported that their aggressiveness caused problems in relating to associates and family members.

Nine of the women felt that athletes should not be tested for anabolic steroid use. If faced with a competition at which testing was to be performed, they would alter their drug use in an attempt to avoid detection.

The participants justified their use of anabolic steroids on several grounds. First, they felt that these drugs were necessary in order to win. Tricker et al. (1989) confirmed this perception and observed that the female bodybuilders in their study generally believed that steroids increased strength and were necessary for them to win.

Second, the side effects, although sometimes undesirable, were acceptable to the participants and their friends, husbands, or significant others. It is likely that women athletes and bodybuilders who use steroids will structure a support network that will approve of the use of these and other performance-enhancing drugs. Both males and females in this network often are lifters or athletes themselves who have used the drugs or at least understand the pressures to use them. However, outsiders to sport, as well as female athletes who have chosen not to use steroids, may look upon these masculinized women as a "freak show" (Dayton, 1990). Finally, participants felt that it was within their individual rights to use anabolic steroids if they wished.

Summary

Anabolic steroid use by women can help to increase muscle strength and size but is associated with multiple adverse side effects, some of them irreversible. Most women athletes choose not to use anabolic steroids, in part because of their masculinizing effects. A few women athletes use steroids because they feel that muscular and strength gains outweigh the risks or the changes that they observe.

References

Anderson, W., & McKeag, D. (1985). *The substance use and abuse habits of college student-athletes* (Research Paper 2). Mission, KS: National Collegiate Athletic Association.

Anderson, W.A., Albrecht, M.A., McKeag, D.B., Hough, D.O., & McGrew, C.A. (1991). A national survey of alcohol and drug use by college athletes. *The Physician and Sportsmedicine*, **19**(2), 91-104.

Bardin, W.C., & Catteral, J. (1981). Testosterone: A major determinant of extragenital sexual dimorphism. *Science*, **211**, 1285-1294.

Dayton, L. (1990, March). What price glory? *Women's Sports & Fitness*, pp. 52-55.

Duchaine, D. (1989). *Underground steroid handbook II*. Venice, CA: HLR Technical Books.

Kochakian, C. (1976). *Anabolic-androgenic steroids*. New York: Springer-Verlag.

Kruskemper, H. (1968). *Anabolic steroids*. New York: Academic Press.

Lindstrom, M., Nilsson, A., Katzman, P., Janzon, L., & Dymling, J. (1990). Use of anabolic-androgenic steroids among body builders—frequency and attitudes. *Journal of Internal Medicine*, **227**, 407-411.

Malarkey, W.B., Strauss, R.H., Leizmen, D.J., Liggett, M.T., & Demers, L.M. (1991). Endocrine effects in women weight lifters self administering testosterone and anabolic steroids. *American Journal of Obstetrics and Gynecology*, **165**, 1385-1390.

Moffatt, R.J., Wallace, M.B., & Sady, S.P. (1990). Effects of anabolic steroids on lipoprotein profiles of female weight lifters. *The Physician and Sportsmedicine*, **18**, 106-115.

Newman, M. (1987). *Elite women athletes survey results.* Center City, MN: Hazelden Research Services.

Spinder, T., Spijkstra, J.J., Van Den Tweel, J.G., Burger, C.W., Van Kessel, H., Hompes, P.G.A., & Gooren, L.J.G. (1989). The effects of long term testosterone administration on pulsatile luteinizing hormone secretion and on ovarian histology in eugonadal female to male transsexual subjects. *Journal of Clinical Endocrinology and Metabolism,* **69,** 151-157.

Strauss, R.H.,Liggett, M.T., & Lanese, R.R. (1985). Anabolic steroid use and perceived effects in ten weight-trained women athletes. *Journal of the American Medical Association,* **253,** 2871-2873.

Tricker, R., O'Neill, M., & Cook, D. (1989). The incidence of anabolic steroid use among competitive bodybuilders. *Journal of Drug Education,* **19,** 313-325.

Voy, R. (1991). *Drugs, sport, and politics.* Champaign, IL: Leisure Press.

Wadler, G., & Hainline, B. (1989). *Drugs and the athlete.* Philadelphia: Davis.

Yen, S., & Jaffee, R. (1978). *Reproductive endocrinology.* Philadelphia: Saunders.

Yesalis, C.E., Buckley, W.A., Anderson, W.A., Wang, M.O., Norwig, I.A., Ott, G., Puffer, I.C., & Strauss, R.H. (1990). Athletes' projections of anabolic steroid use. *Clinical Sports Medicine,* **2,** 155-171.

CHAPTER 8

Psychological Effects of Endogenous Testosterone and Anabolic-Androgenic Steroids

Michael S. Bahrke

"There's no doubt in my mind that when I took the drugs (steroids) I was no longer the same person I was before I took them. And I'm not simply talking about the facial hair and the lower voice. My personality completely changed. I trained harder. I wanted to win more. And I got much more aggressive. There was one woman at the nationals last year who looked at me the wrong way, so I invited her out into the hall."

TAM THOMPSON
"Anabolic Steroids: The Gremlins of Sport,"
Terry Todd, *Journal of Sport History* 14(1): p. 89, 1987

This chapter is adapted from Bahrke, Yesalis, and Wright (1990) by permission; see credits page for more information.

The psychological and behavioral aspects of maleness were noted by Aristotle prior to 300 B.C. (Newerla, 1943) and were studied in numerous uncontrolled experiments up through the 1800s; these experiments sought to demonstrate that the testes contain substances that produce and maintain vitality, strength, energy, and youthfulness (Brown-Sequard, 1889). In the late 1930s, when commercial preparations became available, researchers began to experimentally and clinically explore the effects of purified sex hormones, including effects on mood and mental disorders (Miller, Hubert, & Hamilton, 1938; Salmon & Geist, 1943; Samuels, Henschel, & Keys, 1942; Vest & Howard, 1938). Since that time, a number of literature reviews have reported on these and other effects (Choi, Parrott, & Cowan, 1989; Haupt & Rovere, 1984; Hickson, Ball, & Falduto, 1989; Kochakian, 1976; Kopera, 1985; Kruskemper, 1968; Lamb, 1984; Taylor, 1982; J.D. Wilson, 1988; J.D. Wilson & Griffith, 1980; Wright, 1978, 1980, 1982; Wright & Stone, 1985).

For many years testosterone preparations were rather widely and successfully used in the treatment of involutional psychoses, melancholia, and depression (Altschule & Tillotson, 1948; Ault, Hoctor, & Werner, 1937; Beumont, Bancroft, Beardwood, & Russell, 1972; Burnett, 1963; Danziger & Blank, 1942; Guirdham, 1940; Hamilton, 1937; Heller & Myers, 1944; Itil, 1976; MacMaster & Alamin, 1963; Sansoy, Roy, & Shields, 1971; Tec, 1974; Thomas & Hill, 1940; Vogel, Klaiber, & Broverman, 1985; Werner, 1939, 1943; Werner et al., 1934; Wynn & Landon, 1961). Recently, however, in contrast to these earlier findings, more focused clinical reports have suggested that affective and psychotic syndromes, some of violent proportions, may be associated with the use of anabolic-androgenic steroids in particular individuals (Annitto & Layman, 1980; Baker, 1987; Choi et al., 1989; Conacher & Workman, 1989; Freinhar & Alvarez, 1985; Katz & Pope, 1990; Leckman & Scahill, 1990; Moore, 1988; Pope & Katz, 1987, 1988, 1990). Several cases have been reported wherein defendants alleged that presumed psychological and behavioral effects of anabolic-androgenic steroids significantly influenced the commission of criminal acts (Conacher & Workman, 1989; "Doctor," 1988; "Ex-player's odd behavior," 1988; "The Insanity," 1988; "Killing try," 1988; Lubell, 1989; *Maryland v. Michael D. Williams*, 1986; Moss, 1988). This legal strategy has been identified in the popular press as the "dumbbell defense" ("The insanity," 1988).

The purposes of this chapter are to discuss

- potential mechanisms for some androgen effects on the nervous system,

- the relationship between plasma testosterone levels and aggression in animals and humans,
- the effects of the clinical use of anabolic-androgenic steroids on mood and behavior,
- the relationship of anabolic-androgenic steroid use to behavior and mental health, and
- the major methodological issues involved in assessing the relationship between androgen levels and mood and behavior.

Effects of Anabolic-Androgenic Steroids on the Nervous System

Research has shown anabolic-androgenic steroids to have significant effects on both the development and function of the nervous system. Many years ago, androgens were shown to act directly on the brain (Phoenix, Goy, Gerall, & Young, 1959). These authors suggested that during a male's early development, androgens act to organize neural pathways involved in male behaviors, whereas during adulthood androgens act on differentiated pathways to activate previously organized behaviors. Data from animal studies indicate that both estrogens and androgens act on neural structures that are identical to, or closely associated with, sensory pathways and the ventricular recess organs of the hypothalamus (Stumpf & Sar, 1976). Stumpf and Sar (1976) also reported that androgens selectively stimulate neurons of the somatomotor system and circuits associated with aggression. Itil, Cora, Akpinar, Herrmann, and Patterson (1974) demonstrated quantitatively the physiological correlates of certain previously reported behavioral effects of anabolic-androgenic steroids. These include an increase of mental alertness, elevation of mood, improvement of memory and concentration, and reduction of sensations of fatigue, all of which can be partly related to the "stimulatory" effects of anabolic-androgenic steroids on the central nervous system. Itil et al. (1974) found that electroencephalographic profiles resulting from varying dosages of anabolic-androgenic steroids were very similar to those seen with such psychostimulants as dextroamphetamine and the tricyclic antidepressants. Others (Broverman, Klaiber, Kobayashi, & Vogel, 1968; Klaiber, Broverman, & Kobayashi, 1967; Stenn, Klaiber, Vogel, & Broverman, 1972) have concluded that the adrenergic-like effects of testosterone on brain function are a result of an elevation of the brain's norepinephrine level, which might result from the inhibition of monoamine oxidase activity in the brain. Further speculation indicates that the "heightened" state of behavioral reactivity that facilitates the automatiziation of behavior may well be due to an increased level of norepinephrine in the brain.

Inasmuch as improvements in muscle strength and power can, in part, be accounted for by neural factors, including neurotransmitter levels (Hakkinen & Komi, 1983; Moritani & deVries, 1979), findings that androgens may in some manner modify neural and neuromuscular functions support the concept that these mechanisms (elevated norepinephrine, reduced monoamine levels) play a significant role in the production of ergogenic effects (Alen, Hakkinen, & Komi, 1984; Brooks, 1980; Hakkinen & Alen, 1986; Wilson, 1988).

Plasma Testosterone Levels and Aggression in Animals and Humans

Numerous studies have documented relationships between testosterone levels, dominance, and aggressive behavior in various species of animals including nonhuman primates (Allee, Collias, & Lutherman, 1939; Barfield, Busch, & Wallen, 1972; Bouissou, 1983; Bouissou & Gaudioso, 1982; Hamilton, 1938; Joslyn, 1973; Kurischko & Oettel, 1977; Payne & Swanson, 1973; Rejeski, Brubaker, Herb, Kaplan, & Koritnik, 1988; Rose, Holaday, & Bernstein, 1971; Simon, Whalen, & Tate, 1985; Steklis, Brammer, Raleigh, & McGuire, 1985; Svare, 1983; van de Poll, de Jonge, van Oyen, van Pelt, & de Bruin, 1981; van de Poll, van Zanten, & de Jonge, 1986; Zumpe & Michael, 1985). In general, these and other studies indicate that the animal's level of testosterone, particularly in the prenatal period, but also during puberty and even in adulthood, is important in establishing a biologic readiness for normal, aggressive behavior and in facilitating (in the adult animal) the expression of aggression in "appropriate" social settings. These studies also indicate that both learning and social factors significantly influence the actual expression of aggression in adulthood (Bernstein, Rose, & Gordon, 1974; Rada, Kellner, & Winslow, 1976; Rose, Bernstein, & Gordon, 1975). However, what is not known is the extent to which exposure to testosterone or other anabolic-androgenic steroids at any phase of the life cycle, and particularly during adulthood, is related to altered moods and feelings in humans and to expressions of aggression in humans and even other primates, relative to animals lower in the evolutionary chain.

Fewer studies have assessed the relationship of endogenous or exogenous androgens to aggression or violent behavior in humans (Archer, 1991). In general, this relationship is less clearly established in human research than in animal research for a variety of reasons. First, it is difficult to demonstrate that animals, possibly excluding primates, experience emotional states that are qualitatively similar to human experiences such as euphoria, depression, anger, and others. Second, the effects of sex hormones vary considerably among individuals as well as species. Consequently, conclusions drawn from animal models must be applied cautiously to humans. Lastly, human subjects cannot be subjected to many of the stringent controls and manipulations used in animal research. Nevertheless, a number of studies using human subjects have demonstrated that aggressive behavior and other feelings of hostility are related to endogenous testosterone levels. These investigations, which correlate levels of testosterone with aggressive behavior, have been conducted with incarcerated and nonincarcerated males, and men with genetic differences in testosterone production. Studies have also investigated the effects on behavior of administered testosterone and antiandrogenic agents.

Several studies have examined the relationship between testosterone levels and aggression in adolescents and young adults. Susman and associates have reported on the relationship between hormone levels and emotional dispositions and aggressive attributes for young adolescents (Susman et al., 1985; Susman, Inoff-Germain et al., 1987; Susman, Nottlemann, Inoff-Germain, Dorn, & Chrousos, 1987). The results indicate that a high-for-age hormone level or early timing of puberty generally was related to adverse psychological consequences for boys and girls, with relations being stronger for boys than girls. Udry, Billy, Morris, Groff, and Raj (1985) found that serum testosterone was a strong predictor of sexual motivation and behavior in a sample of 102 boys in Grades 8, 9, and 10. No such relationship, however, could be detected in healthy young adult men (Brown, Monti, & Corriveau, 1978).

Olweus, Mattsson, Schalling, and Low (1980) examined serum testosterone, aggression, physical characteristics, and personality dimensions in 58 typical, healthy 16-year-old adolescent males; the study found a significant association between testosterone and self-reports of physical and verbal aggression, the self-reports mainly reflecting responsiveness to provocation and threat. This finding was supported by Olweus, Mattsson, Schalling, and Low in 1988. Scaramella and Brown (1978) designed a study to examine the relationship between serum testosterone levels and aggressive behaviors in a noncompetitive setting; the subjects were 14 varsity college male hockey players. The authors found a significant positive correlation between serum testosterone and only one of seven aggressive items on their own aggression questionnaire. Elias (1981) measured levels of circulating cortisol, testosterone, and testosterone-binding globulin in 15 male wrestlers in relation to the outcome of wrestling bouts; the study found that concentrations of both cortisol and testosterone increased consistently during wrestling bouts, whereas levels of testosterone-binding globulin dropped. Winners of competitive matches showed significantly greater increases in both hormones than did losers.

Some investigators have examined the relationship of testosterone and mood in adult males. Perskey, Smith, and Basu (1971) determined the plasma testosterone levels and testosterone production rates in a group of

18 healthy young men, 15 healthy older men, and 6 hospitalized dysphoric men. In the younger men, production rate of testosterone was found to be significantly correlated with both the sum of the hostility responses (Total Hostility Score of the Buss-Durkee Hostility Inventory [BDHI]) and the Institute for Personality and Ability Testing (IPAT) Anxiety Scale. Brown and Davis (1975) also found a significant correlation of the BDHI subscale *irritability* with plasma testosterone level in 15 healthy college males. The association between mood and testosterone levels in 20 normal young men was also investigated by Doering et al. (1975), who found only a very weak positive relationship between affect and testosterone. In contrast, Meyer-Bahlburg, Boon, Sharma, and Edwards (1974) found no significant differences in the blood production rates, plasma levels, or urinary levels of androgens in five low-aggression and six high-aggression subjects. Monti, Brown, and Corriveau (1977) likewise failed to find any correlation between aggression and the concentration of circulating testosterone in 101 healthy 20- to 30-year-old males, who displayed a wide range of both testosterone values and BDHI responses.

Testosterone levels and aggression have been examined in other investigations with prisoners (Bradford & McLean, 1984; Dabbs, Frady, Carr, & Besch, 1987; Dabbs, Ruback, Frady, Hopper, & Sgoutas, 1988). Kreuz and Rose (1972) studied levels of plasma testosterone, fighting and verbal aggression in prison, and past criminal behavior in 21 young prisoners; the authors found that although there were significant correlations among psychological inventories, none of the test scales correlated with plasma testosterone, nor did any test scales correlate with fighting behavior. Ehrenkrantz, Bliss, and Sheard (1974) examined plasma testosterone levels in 36 male prisoners, 12 who displayed chronic aggressive behavior, 12 who were socially dominant without physical aggressiveness, and 12 who were neither physically aggressive nor socially dominant. Both the aggressive and the socially dominant groups had significantly higher mean testosterone levels than the nonaggressive group. The aggressive group also had a significantly higher level of testosterone than the non-dominant group, but not significantly higher than the socially dominant group, and the aggressive group's level was higher than those of the other two groups combined. The aggressive group also scored higher than either of the other two groups in the Total Hostility Score of the BDHI. Rada, Laws, and Kellner (1976) also found that within imprisoned sex offenders, a group of 5 violent rapists had significantly higher testosterone levels than 12 child molesters, 47 other "less violent" rapists, or a control group of 48 healthy male prison employees. Schiavi, Theilgaard, Owen, and White (1984) noted a proportionately significant increase in levels of testosterone respectively when subjects were divided into groups of nondelinquents, delinquents convicted of nonviolent crimes, and delinquents convicted of violent crimes. However, the relationship between testosterone level and criminal behavior was not reflected in measures of aggression derived from either psychological interviews or projective tests.

Additional studies have examined the relationship of testosterone to moods other than aggression. Houser (1979) examined the inter- and intrasubject correlations between testosterone and various measures of behavior, affect, and physical discomfort in five young males over a 10-week period and found that a general deterioration of central nervous system motor functioning and a decrease in positive affect were associated with higher testosterone levels. In a study of serum testosterone levels, social status, and mood in male graduate students, Mazur and Lamb (1980) reported that changes in testosterone levels were related to the subject's mood. A study by Tanaka et al. (1989) found that positive mental health and athletic achievement motivation were significantly correlated with higher levels of plasma testosterone.

In summary, several studies have revealed a pattern of association between plasma testosterone and both subjectively perceived aggressive behavior and observed aggressive behavior (Brown & Davis, 1975; Elias, 1981; Olweus et al., 1980; Persky et al., 1971; Scaramella & Brown, 1978). However, the relationships between plasma testosterone and psychometric indices of aggression and hostility have been less consistent (Kreuz & Rose, 1972; Meyer-Bahlburg et al., 1974; Monti et al., 1977; Rada, Laws, & Kellner, 1976; Schiavi et al., 1984). Finally, the other side (and an important consideration) of the question of the relationship of testosterone, mood, and behavior is the extent to which aggressive behavior, successful "expression" of aggression, and nonaggressive success produce higher levels of testosterone (Booth, Shelley, Mazur, Tharp, & Kittok, 1989; Mazur & Lamb, 1980; Salvador, Simon, Suay, & Llorens, 1987; Tanaka et al., 1989). The cause-and-effect relationship between elevated testosterone levels and increased aggressive behavior is unclear.

Effects of Clinical Use of Anabolic-Androgenic Steroids on Mood and Behavior in Patients

Research and anecdotal information suggested some time ago that the use of steroids results in (along with many side effects) various mental disturbances including schizophrenia and manic depression, even though in the mid-1930s estrone was used successfully in both males and females to treat depression and other mental disturbances occurring with menopause and what would now probably be referred to as "andropause."

It is now well known that in excess glucocorticoids can produce emotional instability, ranging from euphoria to suicidal despondency (Hall, 1980). Mental disorders associated with corticosteroid administration have been documented since the early 1950s (Borman & Schmallenberg, 1951;

Brody, 1952; Byyny, 1976; Clark, Bauer, & Cobb, 1952; d'Orban, 1989; Glaser, 1953; Rome & Braceland, 1952; Train & Winkler, 1962), and several literature reviews have related the characteristics of corticosteroid-induced psychiatric disorders (Alcena & Alexopoulos, 1985; Fricchione, Ayyala, & Holmes, 1989; Kaufmann, Kahaner, Peselow, & Gershon, 1982; Lewis & Smith, 1983; Ling, Perry, & Tsuang, 1981). If we consider the structural similarities of cortical and anabolic-androgenic steroids, and their multiple additive, synergistic, and competitive actions, it is not surprising that their administration could result in similar effects on mood and behavior.

Androgens have been used in the treatment of mental disorders for over 50 years. Results from published studies generally indicate positive, rather than negative, effects following androgen therapy in mental (especially depressed) patients (Altschule & Tillotson, 1948; Ault, Hoctor, & Werner, 1937; Barahal, 1938, 1940; Beaumont et al., 1972; Burnett, 1963; Danziger, 1942; Danziger & Black, 1942; Danziger, Schroeder, & Unger, 1944; Davidoff & Goodstone, 1942; Foss, 1937; Guirdham, 1940; Hamilton, 1937; Heller & Myers, 1944; Itil, 1976; Jakobovits, 1970; Kerman, 1943; Lamar, 1940; MacMaster & Alamin, 1963; Palmer, Hastings, & Sherman, 1941; Pardoll & Belinson, 1941; Sands & Chamberlain, 1952; Sansoy et al., 1971; Schmitz, 1937; Schube, McManamy, Trapp, & Houser, 1937; Simonson, Kearns, & Enzer, 1944; Strauss, Sands, Robinson, Tindall, & Stevenson, 1952; Tec, 1974; Thomas & Hill, 1940; Vogel et al., 1985; Werner, 1939, 1943; Werner et al., 1934; Werner, Kohler, Ault, & Hoctor, 1936; Wilson, Prange, & Lara, 1974; Wynn & Landon, 1961; Zeifert, 1942). However, it is unknown whether long-term use of androgens or use of pharmacological doses of androgens by otherwise healthy individuals, particularly adolescents, will result in similar outcomes.

Several studies have examined, with mixed results, the effects of androgen therapy in individuals with androgen deficiencies (Cantrill, Dewis, Large, Newman, & Anderson, 1984; Davidson, Camargo, & Smith, 1979; Franchi, Luisi, & Kicovic, 1978; Franchimont, Kicovic, Mattei, & Roulier, 1978; Gooren, 1987; Luisi & Franchi, 1980; Myhre, Ruvalcaba, Johnson, Thuline, & Kelley, 1970; Nicholls & Anderson, 1982; Nielsen, Johnsen, & Sorensen, 1980; O'Carroll, 1984; O'Carroll & Bancroft, 1985; O'Carroll, Shapiro, & Bancroft, 1985; Salmimies, Kockott, Pirke, Vogt, & Schill, 1982; Skakkebaek, Bancroft, Davidson, & Warner, 1981; Sourial & Fenton, 1988; Wu, Bancroft, Davidson, & Nichol, 1982). Some studies demonstrate significant, positive psychological changes with anabolic-androgenic steroid therapy (Franchi et al., 1978; Franchimont et al., 1978; Luisi & Franchi, 1980; O'Carroll et al., 1985; Skakkebaek et al., 1981), but others do not (Davidson et al., 1979; Salmimies et al., 1982; Wu et al., 1982). However, none of the studies reported adverse or undesired psychological or behavioral effects. Interestingly, five of the six studies that administered oral androgens (Franchi et al., 1978; Franchimont et al., 1978; Luisi & Franchi,

1980; O'Carroll et al., 1985; Skakkebaek et al., 1981) reported improved mood states in subjects following therapy; the two studies that used intramuscular injections of various testostoerone esters (Davidson et al., 1979; Salmimies et al., 1982) found no change. Finally, in a carefully controlled, double-blind crossover comparison of biweekly injections of testosterone esters or placebo in two groups of men with normal testosterone levels, O'Carroll and Bancroft (1984) found no significant change in mood ratings following 12 weeks of treatment.

In addition to the studies that examined the effects of androgen therapy in androgen-deficient males, other studies carried out over the past 2 decades have assessed the contraceptive efficiency of hormonally induced azoospermia in normal men (Burris, Ewing, & Sherins, 1988; Matsumoto, 1988; Schearer et al., 1978). In an investigation conducted by the World Health Organization Task Force on Methods for the Regulation of Male Fertility (1990), 157 of 271 men became azoospermic following weekly testosterone injections and were followed over a 1-year efficacy phase. Although subjects withdrew from the study for several reasons, only three participants reported that they withdrew from the study because of increased aggressiveness and libido resulting from the injections. The authors did not report problems of increased aggressiveness or libido for men who remained in the study.

Although findings of the studies discussed in this section generally indicate positive benefits following androgen therapy in both mental and hypogonadal patients, the psychological and behavioral effects accompanying steroid use by athletes have not been found to be as laudable.

Anabolic-Androgenic Steroid Use, Behavior, and Mental Health

The use of anabolic-androgenic steroids by athletes is associated with many undesirable effects. However, it is quite possible that many of the psychological and behavioral changes attributed to anabolic-androgenic steroid use may have resulted from several years of weight training, or weight training in conjunction with steroid use.

Weight Lifting and Behavior

Very few studies are available that have examined the personality and psychological characteristics of the changes that competitive weight lifters and bodybuilders who do not use anabolic-androgenic steroids may incur as a result of heavy resistance training. Three of the four studies discussed here were conducted before the systematic use of anabolic-androgenic steroids became common; these studies provide us an opportunity to isolate the effects of resistance training on behavior. In a study examining the personalities of track athletes, student pilots, physical education majors, and students enrolled in weight lifting, Henry (1941) found that weight lifters were significantly more introverted, hypersensitive, and hypochondriac, and they felt inferior to other males. Thune (1949), in a study of YMCA weight lifters, reported that a lack of self-confidence or aggressiveness and a desire "to be more manly" were major factors influencing men to participate in a weight-lifting program. In a comparison of 20 weight lifters and 20 non-weight-lifting males, Harlow (1951) found weight lifters to have significantly greater feelings of masculine inadequacy, rejection, dependency, and homosexual tendencies, leading the author to conclude that "weight training seems to be an attempted solution for feelings of masculine inadequacy and inferiority" (p. 322). Freedson, Mihevic, Loucks, and Girandola (1983) found 10 competitive female bodybuilders to be somewhat less anxious, neurotic, depressed, angry, fatigued, and confused and more extroverted, vigorous, and self-motivated than the general population, indicating "good mental health" (p. 89). Unfortunately, Freedson et al. (1983) did not mention whether their subjects were anabolic-androgenic steroid users.

Beyond the few studies examining the personality and psychological alterations that may accompany weight lifting, researchers have little understanding of the extent to which resistance (or other) training may affect or facilitate the expression of aggression. Psychological and behavioral changes, such as increased aggressiveness and irritability, have been reported on an anecdotal basis by athletes who use anabolic-androgenic steroids as well as by their families and friends (Goldman, Bush, & Klatz, 1984; Taylor, 1982, 1987a, 1987b; Wright, 1978, 1982). It is possible, that, as occurs with the use of so many drugs, many of the subjectively perceived psychological and behavioral changes reported by anabolic-androgenic steroid users are a direct result of expectancy, imitation, or role modeling. Observing the actions of other anabolic-androgenic steroid users and athletes may greatly influence the expectations and behaviors of those in the initial and early stages of use. In addition, aggressive or even violent behavior that may be unacceptable outside the athletic environment may be not only fully acceptable but actually encouraged and even required within the weight room or on the playing field.

Psychological Benefits of Anabolic-Androgenic Steroid Use

Several researchers (Brooks, 1980; Ryan, 1981; Wilson & Griffin, 1980) have suggested that some, if not most, of the ergogenic benefits of anabolic-androgenic steroids may derive from their psychological effects. It is possible that anabolic-androgenic steroid use may elevate arousal (Rejeski, Brubaker, Herb, Kaplan, & Manuck, 1988), increase self-confidence and pain threshold (Holzbauer, 1976), and facilitate expression of the all-out physical effort demanded during training and competition in a variety of sports. In the absence of adequate external forces, internal discipline, or social coping skills, these phenomena can lead to expression of aggression at inappropriate times.

Hervey et al. (1976) reported that one value of taking anabolic-androgenic steroids, as expressed by some athletes, lay in the reduction of fatigue during the training season, which allows for more training to be done. Freed, Banks, Longson, and Burley (1975) provided anecdotal or self-reported information that athletes using anabolic-androgenic steroids generally are less easily fatigued, which allows for longer, more frequent, and more intense training sessions. This may be related to the fact that anabolic-androgenic steroids can block and reverse the catabolic effects of glucocorticosteroids that are released during periods of stress including physical exertion (Boone et al., 1990; Kochakian, 1976; Kruskemper, 1968; Williams, 1981). Brooks (1980) suggested that the increases in aggression and energy that the athlete feels may be the result of the neurological changes previously mentioned. In cases in which anabolic-androgenic steroids do improve physical or physiological capacities or performance, the improvement is likely due, to some extent, to increases in training per se as well as to any pharmacological effect.

For the most part, individuals use anabolic-androgenic steroids to significantly improve appearance, performance, or both beyond what is expected from training alone (Catlin & Hatton, 1991). Also, individuals who use anabolic-androgenic steroids appear to believe that higher doses and continued use result in greater gains (Alen & Hakkinen, 1985; Alen, Hakkinen, & Komi, 1984; Alen, Rahkila, Reinila, Reijo, 1987; Alen, Reinila, & Vihko, 1985; Forbes, 1985; Hakkinen & Alen, 1986; Hervey et al., 1976; Kilshaw, Harkness, Hobson, & Smith, 1975). When individuals discontinue using anabolic-androgenic steroids, their size and strength diminish, often very dramatically (Alen & Hakkinen, 1985; Alen, Hakkinen, & Komi, 1984; Alen et al., 1984, 1987; Forbes, 1985; Hakkinen & Alen, 1986). This outcome, as well as any psychological effects of use that serve to create a new body image, improved self-esteem, heightened libido, and general euphoria, is thought to motivate renewed use of anabolic-androgenic steroids (Yesalis, Streit, et al., 1989; Yesalis, Vicary et al., 1990).

Despite these suggestions and self-reports, the literature lacks scientific data supporting the notion that psychological changes (enhanced arousal, confidence, aggression, and motivation) play a primary role in mediating any ergogenic effects of anabolic steroids.

Effects of Anabolic-Androgenic Steroid Use on Mental Health in Athletes

Several studies have examined the side effects of anabolic-androgenic steroids (Annitto & Layman, 1980; Freinhar & Alvarez, 1985; Haupt & Rovere, 1984; Lindstrom, Nilsson, Katzman, Janzon, & Dymling, 1990; Pope & Katz, 1987; Strauss, Ligget, & Lanese, 1985; Strauss, Wright, Finerman, & Catlin, 1983; Tilzey, Heptonstall, & Hamblin, 1981). Currently, the most frequently quoted report concerning the psychological and behavioral effects of anabolic-androgenic steroids is that of Pope and Katz (1988). This report serves as an example of the problems researchers typically encounter when examining the psychological and behavioral effects associated with anabolic-androgenic steroid use. Pope and Katz interviewed 41 steroid users using a structured diagnostic interview. The researchers compared self-reports of various psychiatric syndromes that subjects experienced during anabolic-androgenic steroid use to self-reports about periods of no anabolic-androgenic steroid use. Results indicate that according to DSM-III-R criteria, five subjects (12%) manifested psychotic symptoms, four others (10%) had "subthreshold" or equivocal psychotic symptoms, five subjects (12%) reported manic episodes, and nine subjects (22%) developed full affective syndromes during anabolic-androgenic steroid use. (DSM-III-R refers to the *Diagnostic and Statistical Manual of Mental Disorders*, 1987; see chapter 9.) It is unclear whether these groups were mutually exclusive. None of the 41 subjects recalled adverse effects of anabolic-androgenic steroids sufficient to require medical consultation, and apparently none sought treatment for these mental health disturbances. Pope and Katz did not elaborate on their recruitment of participants, other than to report that subjects were volunteers obtained through advertisements at 38 gymnasiums in the Boston and Santa Monica areas and were paid $25 for a confidential interview; the authors did state that "despite our considerable efforts at recruitment, only a minority of steroid users were willing to be interviewed" (p. 489). Unfortunately, their difficulty in obtaining subjects raises questions about the representativeness of their sample relative to the population of anabolic-androgenic steroid users. Given the vast pool of potential participants, these researchers' difficulty in obtaining volunteers may suggest a low incidence of psychiatric problems among anabolic-androgenic steroid users as well as a basic mistrust of the medical and scientific establishments. It is conceivable that those anabolic-androgenic steroid users who elected to participate in the study were individuals with the greatest severity and frequency of mental disturbance. It is also probably safe to assume that individuals willing to take anabolic-androgenic steroids and other drugs of questionable origin, content, and purity, which have serious legal implications as well as health effects, differ from the population on a wide variety of characteristics, including mental health. Fifteen percent of Pope and Katz's subjects reported past alcohol abuse or dependence, and 32% reported other prior substance abuse or dependence, including use of cannibis (17%) and cocaine (12%). Interpretation of the reports of these subjects must be tempered by the lack of information regarding the extent to which alcohol and other drug use occurred concurrently with anabolic-androgenic steroid use and with psychiatric symptoms and by the absence of knowledge about the interaction of anabolic-androgenic steroids and such drugs of abuse. Seventeen percent of subjects had a first-degree relative with a major affective disorder (somewhat higher than what would be expected; Kaplan & Sadock, 1990), and two subjects reported symptoms of a full affective disorder when not taking steroids. It is difficult to establish the extent to which anabolic-androgenic steroids may have contributed to the psychotic episodes reported by Pope and Katz, and the media have sensationalized these researchers' findings somewhat; it seems likely that with more widespread use of anabolic-androgenic steroids and increased efforts to document such reactions, additional cases will be forthcoming.

In a more recent investigation, Perry, Andersen, and Yates (1990) used two self-report instruments, the Personality Disorder Questionnaire and the Symptom Checklist–90 (SCL-90), as well as a verbal interview based on the National Institutes of Mental Health's Diagnostic Interview Schedule (DIS) to examine mental status changes in 20 competitive and noncompetitive weight lifters who used anabolic-androgenic steroids. In responses to the SCL-90, subjects admitted to increased hostility and aggression, depression, paranoid thoughts, and psychotic features during steroid use. The Personality Disorder Questionnaire revealed that the steroid users displayed more personality disturbances overall compared with a control group of 20 weight lifters who did not use anabolic-androgenic steroids and a sex- and age-matched control group from the local community. Although no individual personality disorder or trait differences were significant between steroid users and the weight-lifter controls, both steroid user and nonsteroid user weight-lifter groups exhibited more flamboyant features (histrionic, narcissistic, antisocial, and borderline) when contrasted to the community controls. The DIS was unable to identify any psychiatric diagnoses that were occurring more frequently in either the weight-lifter control group or the steroid group. No cases of panic disorder, major depressive episode (recurrent), grief reaction, mania (bipolar), or atypical bipolar disorder were found. Interestingly, there were two cases of major depression (single episode) in the controls and one in the steroid users. Alcohol abuse was diagnosed in 65% (13) of the weight-lifter controls, whereas 7 (35%) cases of abuse and 2 (10%) cases of dependence were recognized in the steroid users. Drug abuse was observed in one control and one steroid user, and drug dependence was seen in one of the steroid users. Although this study relied on self-report and interview data only and used a relatively small and local sample, it appears to provide basic knowledge for further research strategies.

Using a series of structured interviews (Structured Clinical Interview for DSM-III-R nonpatient), the Buss Durkee Hostility Inventory, and the SCL-90, Dimeff and Malone (1991) found that psychiatric diagnoses were more common in 45 previous users than 31 current users and 88 nonusers of anabolic-androgenic steroids and that psychiatric disease may either predispose one to or result from anabolic-androgenic steroid use.

As part of an effort to assess physiological and psychological states accompanying anabolic-androgenic steroid use, Bahrke, Wright, Strauss, and Catlin (in press) examined the psychological characteristics and subjectively perceived behavioral and somatic changes accompanying steroid use in 12 current anabolic-androgenic steroid users. The results obtained from the users were compared with results obtained from 14 previous users (no use more recent than 1 month) and 24 nonusers. Although both current and former users reported subjectively perceived changes in enthusiasm, aggression, irritability, insomnia, muscle size, and libido when using anabolic-androgenic steroids, the researchers were unable to confirm these changes in comparison across groups using standardized psychological inventories. The presence of subjectively perceived, anabolic-androgenic steroid–associated behavioral and somatic changes in the absence of significant differences in standard psychological inventory responses illustrates the complexity of these relationships and dictates the need for additional research. The findings of Bahrke et al. (in press) are both compatible with and complementary to anecdotes, case reports, and data from individual psychiatrists. The "negative" findings do not negate the possibility of anabolic-androgenic steroids precipitating aberrant behavior in some users. The general impression, however, is that irritability is slightly increased in many users and that in a few users who are premorbid, anabolic-androgenic steroid use may well be sufficient to "push them over the edge" and contribute to irrational or violent behavior, particularly when these people are using other drugs of abuse (Bahrke, Wright, O'Connor, Strauss, & Catlin, 1990). In an investigation similar to the Bahrke et al. (in press) study, Lefavi, Reeve, and Newland (1990) compared 13 current steroid users with 14 nonusers and 18 former users and concluded that anabolic-androgenic steroids may be associated with more frequent episodes of anger, which are of greater intensity and duration, and more hostile attitudes toward others.

As with corticosteroids (Alcena & Alexopoulos, 1985; Alpert & Seigerman, 1986; Amatruda, Hurst, & D'Esopo, 1965; Byyny, 1976; Dixon & Christy, 1980; Judd, Burrows, & Norman, 1983; Kaufmann et al., 1982), researchers are focusing increasing attention and discussion on the withdrawal effects that athletes encounter when they cease use of anabolic-androgenic steroids (Brower, 1989; Brower, Blow, Beresford, & Fuelling, 1989; Brower, Blow, Eliopulos, & Beresford, 1989; Brower, Blow, Young, & Hill, 1991; Brower, Eliopulos, Blow, Catlin, & Beresford, 1990; Goldman et al., 1984; Hays, Littleton, & Stillner, 1990; Kashkin & Kleber, 1989;

Pope & Katz, 1988; Tennant, Black, & Voy, 1988). Interestingly, many of the same effects attributed to anabolic-androgenic steroid use are alleged to occur following anabolic-androgenic steroid cessation (see chapter 11). Purported withdrawal effects include mood swings, violent behavior, rage, and depression, possibly severe enough to lead to thoughts of suicide. However, these findings must be tempered by the fact that individual responses to different anabolic-androgenic steroids, doses, and lengths of administration likely vary somewhat unpredictably. Further, beyond these initial reports, no study has fully documented a threshold dosage that may produce the effects (mood swings, violent behavior, rage, depression) or a time-course concerning the onset or elimination of these effects once anabolic-androgenic steroid use has been initiated or terminated; these factors may depend, in part, on the length of anabolic-androgenic steroid use, particular desired as well as undesired effects experienced, dosage, and a host of other factors. As Svare (1990) indicated, several critical variables involved in modulating the behavioral effects of androgens in animals, including sex, dose/duration, route of administration, type of androgen, and genotype, must be addressed when researchers examine human anabolic-androgenic steroid abuse. Finally, weight training per se may be addictive in the sense of promoting compulsive, stereotypical, and repetitive behavior to include not only strength training but dieting, drug use, and a host of other lifestyle variables as well.

Major Methodological Issues

As mentioned previously, any attempt to evaluate and summarize the psychological and behavioral effects associated with the use of anabolic-androgenic steroids is complicated by the numerous methodological shortcomings of many of the investigations, including inappropriate sampling strategies; lack of adequate control groups; use of several types, doses, and lengths of administration of anabolic-androgenic steroids; and a variety of techniques used to assess the psychological and behavioral outcomes.

A significant number of studies did not control for or report family or previous personal history of mental illness and aggressive behavior, thereby resulting in a possible selection bias in the study population. In addition, selection of physically or mentally ill persons as subjects raises the question of the generalizability of the findings to otherwise healthy individuals. As McGraw (1990) pointed out, there may be a causal link between traumatic events in individuals' lives and their subsequent decisions to use anabolic-androgenic steroids. Many of the studies discussed here were conducted with small sample sizes, thus reducing the statistical power available to the researchers to detect significant differences. Furthermore, small sample sizes have precluded the examination of steroid effects in additional subgroups such as age, race, gender, educational level, and social class. Small sample size makes it difficult for researchers to control for potential confounding variables using multivariate statistical techniques. Sampling of blood and urine was inconsistent among studies, with respect to timing, and was often unreported. Often multiple samples were not obtained. A number of studies failed to incorporate control groups. Many studies, for ethical and legal reasons, did not randomly assign subjects to treatment, use comparable reference groups, or take advantage of single- or double-blind designs.

All anabolic-androgenic steroids are not the same; significant variation among anabolic-androgenic steroids regarding acute physical effects has been noted (Herrmann & Beach, 1976; Kruskemper, 1968; Williams, 1981), and there is significant individual variation in response to the same androgen and dose (Bardin, Catterall, & Janne, 1990). We must be careful when attempting to generalize the psychological and behavioral effects (findings) from a study that used one type of anabolic-androgenic steroid to another study that used a different steroid. There is also the possibility that adverse reactions may represent toxic responses in some individuals (Kochakian, 1990). Also, while reporting the average steroid dose used, some studies failed to examine or report any dose/response relationship. Even when a report provides dosage, estimating the bioavailability equivalence between oral and injectable anabolic-androgenic steroids is difficult. Moreover, in hypogonadal patients it appears that oral anabolic-androgenic steroids are the only anabolic-androgenic steroids that produce positive mood changes, although the doses of injectable steroids administered in these studies tended to be below those required to restore and maintain normal plasma testosterone levels. In other users (athletes) oral anabolic-androgenic steroids are associated with the adverse psychological changes. Finally, because as much as 50 to 80% or more of the anabolic-androgenic steroids used by athletes may have been obtained from black-market sources (Frankle, Cicero, & Payne, 1984; Yesalis et al., 1988), case reports of individuals who use these drugs must be evaluated accordingly given the absence of knowledge concerning the drugs' actual content.

Defining aggression and assessing aggressive behavior are themselves difficult tasks (Kreuz & Rose, 1972). Because the studies used a variety of psychological inventories, comparing findings between studies is difficult. Some studies used nonstandardized or unpublished inventories; as a result, some of the questionnaires may have been inadequate for detecting behavioral change.

Finally, an overriding concern is the accurate documentation of any change in behavior with anabolic-androgenic steroid use. No studies of an athlete's actual behavior while in athletic competition have been reported. Some studies were unclear regarding how authors determined changes in behavior associated with anabolic-androgenic steroid use. It is possible that some of the behavioral differences reported resulted from the method of data collection: Some investigations relied upon self-reports and other self-defined measures of behavioral change, whereas others used observers and/or interviews to document behavioral changes. Consequently, aggressive feelings that failed to be manifested as aggressive actions may have either gone unrecognized or been overreported.

Summary

Studies have used both prospective and retrospective methods to evaluate the psychological and behavioral effects of anabolic-androgenic steroids. However, statements regarding this topic must remain tentative due to the diversity of study designs and results. Many of the reported behavioral effects have come primarily from studies using a small number of subjects who were administered anabolic-androgenic steroids for a variety of clinical conditions. These studies have found positive or unchanged moods and behavior. Extremely small numbers of athletes have been studied, and we can generalize the findings derived from patient populations to athletes only with caution, particularly because athletes are known to use several drugs concurrently (Frankle et al., 1984) and to use black-market drugs (Buckley et al., 1988; Burkett & Falduto, 1984; Frankle et al., 1984; Windsor & Dumitru, 1989), the content of which may be suspect. And last, the interactive effects of anabolic-androgenic steroids and environmental factors, stress levels, and often drugs of various types (including analgesics, anti-inflammatories, alcohol, and other psychoactive substances) on feelings and behavior remain unresolved in humans.

In summary, the few investigations conducted, primarily in prisoner populations, have shown a significant positive relationship between endogenous testosterone levels and aggressive behavior. However, the extent of the relationship and of the interaction between testosterone and aggression is unknown. Do elevated testosterone levels result in more aggressive behavior, or does more aggressive behavior cause testosterone levels to increase? In addition, what does the interaction of physical activity and an emotionally charged environment have on testosterone production and behavior? Future research will undoubtedly need to examine the positive psychological effects of anabolic-androgenic steroid use, that have occurred in the majority of studies involving patients. There may be significant numbers of individuals whose mental health has been improved through anabolic-androgenic steroid use.

The reports and studies cited in this chapter have raised both medical and legal concerns regarding the psychological and behavioral effects of anabolic-androgenic steroids. Unfortunately, objective evidence documenting the short-term psychological and behavioral changes accompanying and following anabolic-androgenic steroid use by athletes is extremely limited and inconclusive. As indicated, many of the studies in this area suffer from methodological inadequacies. As several researchers have pointed out (Cicero & O'Connor, 1990; Yesalis, Anderson, Buckley, & Wright, 1990; Yesalis, Vicary et al., 1990; Yesalis, Wright, & Bahrke, 1989; Yesalis, Wright, & Lombardo, 1989) extremely little is known about the long-term health impact of anabolic-androgenic steroids and their interactions with other drugs, including drugs of abuse. Consequently, the need for much additional research is strongly indicated.

Although some athletes and coaches believe that anabolic-androgenic steroids exert a positive effect by enhancing performance through altered psychological states, others point out the potential negative effects of violent and aggressive behavior. With present estimates of a million or more anabolic-androgenic steroid users in the United States, a tiny percentage of anabolic-androgenic steroid–using athletes appear to experience mental disturbances that result in their seeking clinical treatment, and of those who do, some may already suffer from existing mental health or other substance-abuse problems. At this point a cause-effect relationship has yet to be established. Moreover, of the seemingly small population of individuals who do experience significant psychological and behavioral changes, most apparently recover without legal or other problems when they stop using androgens.

References

Alcena, V., & Alexopoulos, G.S. (1985). Ulcerative colitis in association with chronic paranoid schizophrenia: A review of steroid-induced psychiatric disorders. *Journal of Clinical Gastroenterology*, **7**(5), 400-404.

Alen, M., & Hakkinen, K. (1985). Physical health and fitness of an elite bodybuilder during 1 year of self-administration of testosterone and anabolic steroids: A case study. *International Journal of Sports Medicine*, **6**, 24-29.

Alen, M., Hakkinen, K., & Komi, P.V. (1984). Changes in neuromuscular and muscle fiber characteristics of elite power athletes self-administering androgenic and anabolic steroids. *Acta Physiologica Scandinavica*, **122**, 535-544.

Alen, M., Rahkila, P., Reinila, M., & Reijo, V. (1987). Androgenic-anabolic steroids effects on serum thyroid, pituitary and steroid hormones in athletes. *American Journal of Sports Medicine*, **15**, 357-361.

Alen, M., Reinhila, M., & Vihko, R. (1985). Response of serum hormones to androgen administration in power athletes. *Medicine and Science in Sports and Exercise*, **17**(3), 354-359.

Allee, W.C., Collias, N.E., & Lutherman, C.Z. (1939). Modification of the social order in flocks of hens by the injection of testosterone propionate. *Physiological Zoology*, **12**(4), 412-440.

Alpert, E., & Seigerman, C. (1986). Steroid withdrawal psychosis in a patient with closed head injury. *Archives of Physical Medicine and Rehabilitation, 67*, 766-769.

Altschule, M.D., & Tillotson, K.J. (1948). The use of testosterone in the treatment of depressions. *New England Journal of Medicine, 239*(17), 1036-1038.

Amatruda, T.T., Hurst, M.M., & D'Esopo, N.D. (1965). Certain endocrine and metabolic facets of the steroid withdrawal syndrome. *Journal of Clinical Endocrinology and Metabolism, 25*, 1207-1217.

Annitto, W.J., & Layman, W.A. (1980). Anabolic steroids and acute schizophrenic episode. *Journal of Clinical Psychiatry, 41*(4), 143-144.

Archer, J. (1991). The influence of testosterone on human aggression. *British Journal of Psychology, 82*, 1-28.

Ault, C.C., Hoctor, E.F., & Werner, A.A. (1937). Theelin therapy in the psychoses. *Journal of the American Medical Association, 109*, 1786-1788.

Bahrke, M.S., Wright, J.E., O'Connor, J.S., Strauss, R.H., & Catlin, D.H. (1990). Selected psychological characteristics of anabolic-androgenic steroid users. *New England Journal of Medicine, 323*(12), 834-835.

Bahrke, M.S., Wright, J.E., Strauss, R.H., & Catlin, D.H. (in press). Psychological moods and subjectively-perceived behavioral and somatic changes accompanying anabolic-androgenic steroid usage. *American Journal of Sports Medicine.*

Barahal, H.S. (1938). Testosterone in male involutional melancholia. *Psychiatric Quarterly, 12*, 743-749.

Barahal, H.S. (1940). Testosterone in psychotic male homosexuals. *Psychiatric Quarterly, 14*, 319-330.

Bardin, C.W., Catterall, J.F., & Janne, O.A. (1990). The androgen-induced phenotype. In G.C. Lin & L. Erinoff (Eds.), *Anabolic steroid abuse* (NIDA Research Monograph) (pp. 131-141). Rockville, MD: National Institute on Drug Abuse.

Barfield, R.J., Busch, D.E., & Wallen, K. (1972). Gonadal influence on agonistic behavior in the male domestic rat. *Hormones and Behavior, 3*, 247-259.

Barker, S. (1987). Oxymetholone and aggression. *British Journal of Psychiatry, 151*, 564.

Bernstein, I.S., Rose, R.M., & Gordon, T.P. (1974). Behavioral and environmental events influencing primate testosterone levels. *Journal of Human Evolution, 3*, 517-525.

Beumont, P.J.V., Bancroft, J.H.J., Beardwood, C.J., & Russell, G.F. (1972). Behavioural changes after treatment with testosterone: Case report. *Psychological Medicine, 2*, 70-72.

Boone, J.B., Lambert, C.P., Flynn, M.G., Michaud, T.J., Rodriguez-Zayas, J.A., & Andres, F.F. (1990). Resistance exercise effects on plasma cortisol, testosterone and creatine kinase activity in anabolic-androgenic steroid users. *International Journal of Sport Medicine, 11*(4), 293-297.

Booth, A., Shelley, G., Mazur, A., Tharp, G., & Kittok, R. (1989). Testosterone, and winning and losing in human competition. *Hormones and Behavior, 23*, 556-571.

Borman, M.C., & Schmallenberg, H.C. (1951). Suicide following cortisone treatment. *Journal of the American Medical Association*, **146**, 337-338.

Bouissou, M.F. (1983). Androgens, aggressive behaviour and social relationships in higher mammals. *Hormone Research*, **18**, 43-61.

Bouissou, M.F., & Gaudioso, V. (1982). Effect of early androgen treatment on subsequent social behavior in heifers. *Hormones and Behavior*, **16**, 132-146.

Bradford, J.M.W., & McLean, D. (1984). Sexual offenders, violence and testosterone: A clinical study. *Canadian Journal of Psychiatry*, **29**, 335-343.

Brody, S. (1952). Psychiatric observations in patients treated with cortisone and ACTH. *Psychosomatic Medicine*, **14**, 94-103.

Brooks, R.V. (1980). Anabolic steroids and athletes. *The Physician and Sportsmedicine*, **8**(3), 161-163.

Broverman, D.M., Klaiber, E.L., Kobayashi, Y., & Vogel, W. (1968). Roles of activation and inhibition in sex differences in cognitive abilities. *Psychological Reviews*, **75**, 23-50.

Brower, K.J. (1989). Rehabilitation for anabolic-androgenic steroid dependence. *Clinical Sports Medicine*, **1**, 171-181.

Brower, K.J., Blow, F.C., Beresford, T.P., & Fuelling, C. (1989). Anabolic-androgenic steroid dependence. *Journal of Clinical Psychiatry*, **50**(1), 31-33.

Brower, K.J., Blow, F.C., Eliopulos, G.A., & Beresford, T.P. (1989). Anabolic androgenic steroids and suicide. *American Journal of Psychiatry*, **146**(8), 1075.

Brower, K.J., Blow, F.C., Young, J.P., & Hill, E.M. (1991). Symptoms and correlates of anabolic-androgenic steroid dependence. *British Journal of Addiction*, **86**, 759-768.

Brower, K.J., Eliopulos, G.A., Blow, F.C., Catlin, D.H., & Beresford, T.P. (1990). Evidence for physical and psychological dependence on anabolic-androgenic steroids in eight weight lifters. *American Journal of Psychiatry*, **147**(4), 510-512.

Brown, W.A., & Davis, G.H. (1975). Serum testosterone and irritability in man. *Psychosomatic Medicine*, **37**(1), 87.

Brown, W.A., Monti, P.M., & Corriveau, D.P. (1978). Serum testosterone and sexual activity and interest in men. *Archives of Sexual Behavior*, **7**, 97-103.

Brown-Sequard, E. (1889). The effects produced on man by subcutaneous injections of a liquid obtained from the testicles of animals. *Lancet*, **2**, 105-107.

Buckley, W.E., Yesalis, C.E., Friedl, K.E., Anderson, W.A., Streit, A.L., & Wright, J.E. (1988). Estimated prevalence of anabolic steroid use among male high school seniors. *Journal of the American Medical Association*, **260**(23), 3441-3445.

Burkett, L.N., & Falduto, M.T. (1984). Steroid use by athletes in a metropolitan area. *The Physician and Sportsmedicine, 12*(8), 69-74.

Burnett, P.C. (1963). A steroidal pyrazole as an anabolic agent in the treatment of geriatric mental patients. *Journal of the American Geriatric Society, 11*, 979-982.

Burris, A.S., Ewing, L.L., & Sherins, R.J. (1988). Initial trial of slow-release testosterone microspheres in hypogonadal men. *Fertility and Sterility, 50*, 493-497.

Byyny, R.L. (1976). Withdrawal from glucocorticoid therapy. *New England Journal of Medicine, 295*(1), 30-32.

Cantrill, J.A., Dewis, P., Large, D.M., Newman, M., & Anderson, D.C. (1984). Which testosterone replacement therapy? *Clinical Endocrinology, 21*, 97-107.

Catlin, D.H., & Hatton, C.K. (1991). Use and abuse of anabolic and other drugs for athletic enhancement. *Advances in Internal Medicine, 36*, 399-424.

Choi, P.Y.L., Parrott, A.C., & Cowan, D. (1989). Adverse behavioural effects of anabolic steroids in athletes: A brief review. *Clinical Sports Medicine, 1*, 183-187.

Cicero, T.J., & O'Connor, L.H. (1990). Abuse liability of anabolic steroids and their possible role in the abuse of alcohol, morphine and other substances. In G.C. Lin & L. Erinoff (Eds.), *Anabolic steroid abuse* (NIDA Research Monograph) (pp. 1-28). Rockville, MD: National Institute on Drug Abuse.

Clark, L.D., Bauer, W., & Cobb, S. (1952). Preliminary observations on mental disturbances occurring in patients under therapy with cortisone and ACTH. *New England Journal of Medicine, 246*, 205-216.

Conacher, G.N., & Workman, D.G. (1989). Violent crime possibly associated with anabolic steroid use. *American Journal of Psychiatry, 146*(5), 679.

Dabbs, J.M., Frady, R.L., Carr, T.S., & Besch, N.F. (1987). Saliva testosterone and criminal violence in young adult prison inmates. *Psychosomatic Medicine, 49*(2), 174-182.

Dabbs, J.M., Ruback, R.B., Frady, R.L., Hopper, C.H., & Sgoutas, D.S. (1988). Saliva testosterone and criminal violence among women. *Personality and Individual Differences, 9*(2), 269-275.

Danziger, L. (1942). Estrogen therapy of agitated depressions associated with the menopause. *Archives of Neurology and Psychiatry, 47*, 305-313.

Danziger, L., & Blank, H.R. (1942). Androgen therapy of agitated depressions in the male. *Medical Annals of the District of Columbia, 11*, 181-183.

Danziger, L., Schroeder, H.T., & Unger, A.A. (1944). Androgen therapy for involutional melancholia. *Archives of Neurology and Psychiatry, 51*, 457-461.

Davidoff, E., & Goodstone, G.L. (1942). Use of testosterone propionate in treatment of involutional psychosis in the male. *Archives of Neurology and Psychiatry*, **48**, 811-817.

Davidson, J.M., Camargo, C.A., & Smith, E.R. (1979). Effects of androgen on sexual behavior in hypogonadal men. *Journal of Clinical Endocrinology and Metabolism*, **48**(6), 955-958.

Dimeff, R., & Malone, D. (1991). Psychiatric disorders in weightlifters using anabolic steroids. *Medicine and Science in Sports and Exercise*, **23**(2) (Suppl.), S18.

Dixon, R.B., & Christy, N.P. (1980). On the various forms of corticosteroid withdrawal syndrome. *American Journal of Medicine*, **68**, 224-230.

Doctor: Steroid rage led to killing. (1988, June 2). *Sun-Sentinel* (Ft. Lauderdale, FL).

Doering, C.H., Brodie, K.M., Kraemer, H.C., Moos, R.H., Becker, H.B., & Hamburg, D.A. (1975). Negative affect and plasma testosterone: A longitudinal study. *Psychosomatic Medicine*, **37**(6), 484-491.

d'Orban, P.T. (1989). Steroid-induced psychosis. *Lancet*, **2**, 694.

Ehrenkrantz, J.E., Bliss, E., & Sheard, M.H. (1974). Plasma testosterone: Correlation with aggressive behavior and social dominance in man. *Psychosomatic Medicine*, **36**(6), 469-475.

Elias, M. (1981). Serum cholesterol, testosterone, and testosterone-binding globulin responses to competitive fighting in human males. *Aggressive Behavior*, **7**, 215-224.

Ex-player's odd behavior due to steroid use, doctor says. (1988, February 14). *Indianapolis Star*, p. B4.

Forbes, G.B. (1985). The effect of anabolic steroids on lean body mass: The dose response curve. *Metabolism*, **34**, 571-573.

Foss, G.L. (1937). Effect of testosterone propionate on a post-pubertal eunuch. *Lancet*, **2**, 1301-1309.

Franchi, F., Luisi, M., & Kicovic, P.M. (1978). Long-term study of oral testosterone undecanoate in hypogonadal males. *International Journal of Andrology*, **1**, 270-278.

Franchimont, P., Kicovic, P.M., Mattei, A., & Roulier, R. (1978). Effects of oral testosterone undecanoate in hypogonadal male patients. *Clinical Endocrinology*, **9**, 313-320.

Frankle, M.A., Cicero, G.J., & Payne, J. (1984). Use of androgenic anabolic steroids by athletes. *Journal of the American Medical Association*, **252**(4), 482.

Freed, D.L., Banks, A.J., Longson, D., & Burley, D.M. (1975). Anabolic steroids in athletics: Crossover double-blind trial on weightlifters. *British Medical Journal*, **2**, 471-473.

Freedson, P.S., Mihevic, P.M., Loucks, A.B., & Girandola, R.N. (1983). Physique, body composition, and psychological characteristics of competitive female body builders. *The Physician and Sportsmedicine*, **11**(5), 85-93.

Freinhar, J.P., & Alvarez, W. (1985). Androgen-induced hypomania. *Journal of Clinical Psychiatry, 46*(8), 354-355.

Fricchione, G., Ayyala, M., & Holmes, V.F. (1989). Steroid withdrawal psychiatric syndromes. *Annals of Clinical Psychiatry, 1*(2), 99-108.

Glaser, G.H. (1953). Psychotic reactions induced by corticotropin (ACTH) and cortisone. *Psychosomatic Medicine, 15*(4), 289-291.

Goldman, B., Bush, P., & Klatz, R. (1984). *Death in the locker room: Steroids and sports.* South Bend, IN: Icarus Press.

Gooren, L.J.G. (1987). Androgen level and sex functions in testosterone-treated hypogonadal men. *Archives of Sexual Behavior, 16*(6), 463-473.

Guirdham, A. (1940). Treatment of mental disorders with male sex hormone. *British Medical Journal, 1*, 10-12.

Hakkinen, K., & Alen, M. (1986). Physiological performance, serum hormones, enzymes and lipids of an elite power athlete during training with and without androgens and during prolonged detraining. *Journal of Sports Medicine, 26*, 92-100.

Hakkinen, K., & Komi, P.V. (1983). Electromyographic changes during strength training and detraining. *Medicine and Science in Sports and Exercise, 15*(6), 455-460.

Hall, R.C.W. (1980). *Psychiatric presentations of medical illness.* New York: Medical and Scientific Books.

Hamilton, J.B. (1937). Treatment of sexual underdevelopment with synthetic male hormone substance. *Endocrinology, 21*, 649-654.

Hamilton, J.B. (1938). Precocious masculine behavior following administration of synthetic male hormone substance. *Endocrinology, 23*, 53-57.

Harlow, R.G. (1951). Masculine inadequacy and compensatory development of physique. *Journal of Personality, 19*, 312-323.

Haupt, H.A., & Rovere, G.D. (1984). Anabolic steroids: A review of the literature. *American Journal of Sports Medicine, 12*(6), 469-484.

Hays, L.R., Littleton, S., & Stillner, V. (1990). Anabolic steroid dependence. *American Journal of Psychiatry, 147*(1), 122.

Heller, C.G., & Myers, G.B. (1944). The male climacteric, its symptomatology, diagnosis and treatment. *Journal of the American Medical Association, 126*(8), 472-477.

Henry, F. (1941). Personality differences in athletes and physical education and aviation students. *Psychological Bulletin, 38*, 745.

Herrmann, W.M., & Beach, R.C. (1976). Psychotropic effects of androgens: A review of clinical observations and new human experimental findings. *Pharmakopsychologie, 9*, 205-219.

Hervey, G.R., Hutchinson, I., Knibbs, A.V., Burkinshaw, L., Jones, P.R.M., Norgan, N.G., & Levell, M.J. (1976). "Anabolic" effects of methandienone in men undergoing athletic training. *Lancet, 2*, 699-702.

Hickson, R.C., Ball, K.L., & Falduto, M.T. (1989). Adverse effects of anabolic steroids. *Medical Toxicology and Adverse Drug Experience, 4*(4), 254-271.

Holzbauer, M. (1976). Physiological aspects of steroids with anaesthetic properties. *Medical Biology*, **54**, 227-242.

Houser, B.B. (1979). An investigation of the correlation between hormonal levels in males and mood, behavior and physical discomfort. *Hormones and Behavior*, **12**, 185-197.

The insanity of steroid abuse. (1988, May 23). *Newsweek*, p. 75.

Itil, T.M. (1976). The neurophysiological models in the development of psychotropic hormones. In T.M. Itil, G. Laudahn, & W. Hermann (Eds.), *Psychotropic action of hormones* (pp. 53-77). New York: Spectrum.

Itil, T.M., Cora, R., Akpinar, S., Herrmann, W.M., & Patterson, C.J. (1974). "Psychotropic" action of sex hormones: Computerized EEG in establishing the immediate CNS effects of steroid hormones. *Current Therapeutic Research*, **16**(11), 1147-1170.

Jakobovits, T. (1970). The treatment of impotence with methyltestosterone thyroid (100 patients—double blind study). *Fertility and Sterility*, **21**(1), 32-35.

Joslyn, W.D. (1973). Androgen-induced social dominance in infant female rhesus monkeys. *Journal of Child Psychology and Psychiatry*, **14**, 137-145.

Judd, F.K., Burrows, G.D., & Norman, T.R. (1983). Psychosis after withdrawal of steroid therapy. *Medical Journal of Australia*, **2**, 350-351.

Kaplan, H.I., & Sadock, B.J. (1990). *Pocket handbook of psychiatry* (6th ed.). Baltimore: Williams & Wilkins.

Kashkin, K.B., & Kleber, H.D. (1989). Hooked on hormones? An anabolic steroid addiction hypothesis. *Journal of the American Medical Association*, **262**(22), 3166-3170.

Katz, D.L., & Pope, H.G. (1990). Anabolic-androgenic steroid-induced mental status changes. In G.C. Lin & L. Erinoff (Eds.), *Anabolic steroid abuse* (NIDA Research Monograph) (pp. 215-223). Rockville, MD: National Institute on Drug Abuse.

Kaufmann, M., Kahaner, K., Peselow, E.D., & Gershon, S. (1982). Steroid psychoses: Case report and brief overview. *Journal of Clinical Psychiatry*, **43**(2), 75-76.

Kerman, E.F. (1943). Testosterone therapy of involutional psychosis. *Archives of Neurology and Psychiatry*, **49**, 306-307.

Killing try is blamed on drugs. (1988, June 25). *Roanoke (VA) Times*, pp. 3-5.

Kilshaw, B.H., Harkness, R.A., Hobson, B.M., & Smith, A.W.M. (1975). The effects of large doses of the anabolic steroid, methandienone, on an athlete. *Clinical Endocrinology*, **4**, 537-541.

Klaiber, E.L., Broverman, D.M., & Kobayashi, Y. (1967). The automatization cognitive style, androgens, and monoamine oxidase. *Psychopharmacologia*, **11**, 320-336.

Kochakian, C.D. (Ed.) (1976). *Anabolic-androgenic steroids*. New York: Springer-Verlag.

Kochakian, C.D. (1990). History of anabolic-androgenic steroids. In G.C. Lin & L. Erinoff (Eds.), *Anabolic steroid abuse* (NIDA Research Monograph) (pp. 25-29). Rockville, MD: National Institute on Drug Abuse.

Kopera, H. (1985). The history of anabolic steroids and a review of clinical experience with anabolic steroids. *Acta Endocrinologica,* **110**(Suppl. 271), 11-18.

Kreuz, L.E., & Rose, R.M. (1972). Assessment of aggressive behavior and plasma testosterone in a young criminal population. *Psychosomatic Medicine,* **34**(4), 321-332.

Kruskemper, H. (1968). *Anabolic steroids.* New York: Academic Press.

Kurischko, A., & Oettel, M. (1977). Androgen-dependent fighting behavior in male mice. *Endokrinologie,* **70,** 1-5.

Lamar, C.P. (1940). Clinical endocrinology of the male with especial reference to the male climacteric. *Journal of the Florida Medical Association,* **26**(8), 398-404.

Lamb, D.R.. (1984). Anabolic steroids in athletics: How well do they work and how dangerous are they? *American Journal of Sports Medicine,* **12**(1), 31-38.

Leckman, J.F., & Scahill, L. (1990). Possible exacerbation of tics by androgenic steroids. *New England Journal of Medicine,* **322**(23), 1674.

Lefavi, R.G., Reeve, T.G., & Newland, M.C. (1990). Relationship between anabolic steroid use and selected psychological parameters in male bodybuilders. *Journal of Sport Behavior,* **13**(3), 157-166.

Lewis, D.A., & Smith, R.E. (1983). Steroid-induced psychiatric syndromes. *Journal of Affective Disorders,* **5,** 319-322.

Ling, M.H.M., Perry, P.J., & Tsuang, M.T. (1981). Side effects of corticosteroid therapy: Psychiatric aspects. *Archives of General Psychiatry,* **38,** 471-477.

Lubell, A. (1989). Does steroid abuse cause or excuse violence? *The Physician and Sportsmedicine,* **17**(2), 176-185.

Luisi, M., & Franchi, F. (1980). Double-blind group comparative study of testosterone undecanoate and mesterolone in hypogonadal male patients. *Journal of Endocrinology Investigations,* **3,** 305-308.

MacMaster, D.R., & Alamin, K. (1963). Treatment of severe weight loss with methandrostenolone—a less virilizing anabolic agent. *American Journal of Psychiatry,* **120,** 179-180.

Maryland v. Michael David Williams. (1986, April). Circuit Court record for St. Mary's County, pp. 5630-5635.

Matsumoto, A.M. (1988). Is high dosage testosterone an effective male contraceptive agent? *Fertility and Sterility,* **50,** 324-328.

Mazur, A., & Lamb, T.A. (1980). Testosterone, status, and mood in human males. *Hormones and Behavior,* **14,** 236-246.

McGraw, J.M. (1990). The psychology of anabolic steroid use. *Journal of Clinical Psychiatry,* **51**(6), 260.

Meyer-Bahlburg, H.F.L., Boon, D.A., Sharma, M., & Edwards, J.A. (1974). Aggressiveness and testosterone measures in man. *Psychosomatic Medicine*, **36**(3), 269-274.

Miller, N.E., Hubert, G., & Hamilton, J.B. (1938). Mental and behavioral changes following male hormone treatment of adult castration, hypogonadism and psychic impotence. *Proceedings of the Society for Experimental Biology and Medicine*, **38**, 538-540.

Monti, P.M., Brown, W.A., & Corriveau, D.P. (1977). Testosterone and components of aggressive and sexual behavior in man. *American Journal of Psychiatry*, **134**(6), 692-694.

Moore, W.V. (1988). Anabolic steroid use in adolescence. *Journal of the American Medical Association*, **260**(23), 3484-3486.

Moritani, T., & deVries, H.A. (1979). Neural factors versus hypertrophy in the time course of muscle strength gain. *American Journal of Physical Medicine*, **58**, 115-130.

Moss, D.C. (1988, October 1). And now the steroid defense? *American Bar Association Journal*, pp. 22-24.

Myhre, S.A., Ruvalcaba, R.H.A., Johnson, H.R., Thuline, H.C., & Kelley, V.C. (1970). The effects of testosterone treatment in Klinefelter's syndrome. *Journal of Pediatrics*, **76**(2), 267-276.

Newerla, G.J. (1943). The history of the discovery and isolation of the male hormone. *New England Journal of Medicine*, **228**(2), 39-47.

Nicholls, D.P., & Anderson, D.C. (1982). Clinical aspects of androgen deficiency in men. *Andrologia*, **14**(5), 379-388.

Nielsen, J., Johnsen, S.G., & Sorensen, K. (1980). Follow-up 10 years later of 34 Klinefelter males with karyotype 47, XXY and 16 hypogonadal males with karyotype 46, XY. *Psychological Medicine*, **10**, 345-352.

O'Carroll, R.E. (1984). Androgen administration to hypogonadal and eugonadal men—effects on measures of sensation seeking, personality, and spatial ability. *Personality and Individual Differences*, **5**(5), 595-598.

O'Carroll, R., & Bancroft, J. (1984). Testosterone therapy for low sexual interest and erectile dysfunction in men: A controlled study. *British Journal of Psychiatry*, **145**, 146-151.

O'Carroll, R.E., & Bancroft, J. (1985). Androgens and aggression in man: A controlled case study. *Aggressive Behavior*, **2**, 1-7.

O'Carroll, R., Shapiro, C., & Bancroft, J. (1985). Androgens, behavior and nocturnal erection in hypogonadal men: The effects of varying the replacement dose. *Clinical Endocrinology*, **23**, 527-538.

Olweus, D.O., Mattsson, A., Schalling, D., & Low, H. (1980). Testosterone, aggression, physical and personality dimensions in normal adolescent males. *Psychosomatic Medicine*, **42**, 253-269.

Olweus, D.O., Mattsson, A., Schalling, D., & Low, H. (1988). Circulating testosterone levels and aggression in adolescent males: A causal analysis. *Psychosomatic Medicine*, **50**, 261-272.

Palmer, H.D., Hastings, D.W., & Sherman, S.H. (1941). Therapy in involutional melancholia. *American Journal of Psychiatry*, **97**, 1086-1115.

Pardoll, D.H., & Belinson, L. (1941). Androgen therapy in psychosis: Effect of testosterone propionate in male involutional psychotics. *Journal of Clinical Endocrinology*, **1**, 138-141.

Payne, A.P., & Swanson, H.H. (1973). The effects of neonatal androgen administration on the aggression and related behavior of golden hamsters during interactions with females. *Journal of Endocrinology*, **58**, 627-636.

Perry, P.J., Andersen, K.H., & Yates, W.R. (1990). Illicit anabolic steroid use in athletes. *American Journal of Sports Medicine*, **18**(4), 422-428.

Persky, H., Smith, K.D., & Basu, G.K. (1971). Relation of psychologic measures of aggression and hostility to testosterone production in man. *Psychosomatic Medicine*, **33**(3), 265-277.

Phoenix, C.H., Goy, R.W., Gerall, A.A., & Young, W.C. (1959). Organizing action of prenatally administered testosterone propionate on the tissues mediating mating behavior in the female guinea pig. *Endocrinology*, **65**, 369-382.

Pope, H.G., & Katz, D.L. (1987). Bodybuilder's psychosis. *Lancet*, **1**, 863.

Pope, H.G., & Katz, D.L. (1988). Affective and psychotic symptoms associated with anabolic steroid use. *American Journal of Psychiatry*, **145**(4), 487-490.

Pope, H.G., & Katz, D.L. (1990). Homicide and near-homicide by anabolic steroid users. *Journal of Clinical Psychiatry*, **51**, 28-31.

Rada, R.T., Kellner, R., & Winslow, W.W. (1976). Plasma testosterone and aggressive behavior. *Psychosomatics*, **17**, 138-141.

Rada, R.T., Laws, D.R., & Kellner, R. (1976). Plasma testosterone levels in the rapist. *Psychosomatic Medicine*, **38**(4), 257-268.

Rejeski, W.J., Brubaker, P.H., Herb, R.A., Kaplan, J.R., & Koritnik, D. (1988). Anabolic steroids and aggressive behavior in cynomolgus monkeys. *Journal of Behavioral Medicine*, **11**(1), 95-105.

Rejeski, W.J., Brubaker, P.H., Herb, R.A., Kaplan, J.R., & Manuck, S.B. (1988). The role of anabolic steroids on baseline and stress heart rate in cynomolgus monkeys. *Health Psychology*, **7**(4), 299-307.

Rome, H.P., & Braceland, F.J. (1952). Psychological response to corticotropin, cortisone, and related steroid substances. *Journal of the American Medical Association*, **148**(1), 27-30.

Rose, R.M., Bernstein, I.S., & Gordon, T.P. (1975). Consequences of social conflict on plasma testosterone levels in rhesus monkeys. *Psychosomatic Medicine*, **37**(1), 50-61.

Rose, R.M., Holaday, J.W., & Bernstein, I.S. (1971). Plasma testosterone, dominance rank and aggressive behaviour in male rhesus monkeys. *Nature*, **231**, 366-368.

Ryan, A.J. (1981). Anabolic steroids are fool's gold. *Federation Proceedings*, **40**, 2682-2688.

Salmimies, P., Kockott, G., Pirke, K.M., Vogt, H.J., & Schill, W.B. (1982). Effects of testosterone replacement on sexual behavior in hypogonadal men. *Archives of Sexual Behavior*, **11**(4), 345-353.

Salmon, U.J., & Geist, S.H. (1943). Effects of androgens upon libido in women. *Journal of American Endocrinology*, **3**, 235-238.

Salvador, A., Simon, V., Suay, F., & Llorens, L. (1987). Testosterone and cortisol responses to competitive fighting in human males. *Aggressive Behavior*, **13**, 9-13.

Samuels, L.T., Henschel, A.F., & Keys, A. (1942). Influence of methyl testosterone on muscular work and creatine metabolism in normal young men. *Journal of Clinical Endocrinology*, **2**, 649-654.

Sands, D.E., & Chamberlain, G.H.A. (1952). Treatment of inadequate personality in juveniles by dehydroisoandrosterone: Preliminary report. *British Medical Journal*, **2**, 66-68.

Sansoy, O.M., Roy, A.N., & Shields, L.M. (1971). Anabolic action and side effects of oxandrolone in 34 mental patients. *Geriatrics*, **26**, 139-143.

Scaramella, T.J., & Brown, W.A. (1978). Serum testosterone and aggressiveness in hockey players. *Psychomatic Medicine*, **40**(3), 262-265.

Schearer, S.B., Alvarez-Sanchez, F., Anselmo, J., Brenner, P., Coutino, E., Latham-Faundes, A., Frick, J., Heinild, B., & Johansson, E.D.B. (1978). Hormonal contraception for men. *International Journal of Andrology*, (Suppl. 2), 680-712.

Schiavi, R.C., Theilgaard, A., Owen, D.R., & White, D. (1984). Sex chromosome anomalies, hormones, and aggressivity. *Archives of General Psychiatry*, **41**, 93-99.

Schmitz, G. (1937). Erfahrungen mit dem nuen synthetischen testeshormonpraparat "Perandren." *Deutsche Medizinische Wochenschrift*, **63**, 230-231.

Schube, P.G., McManamy, M.C., Trapp, C.E., & Houser, G.F. (1937). Involutional melancholia: Treatment with theelin. *Archives of Neurology and Psychiatry*, **38**, 505-512.

Simon, N.G., Whalen, R.E., & Tate, M.P. (1985). Induction of male-typical aggression by androgens but not by estrogens in adult female mice. *Hormones and Behavior*, **19**, 204-212.

Simonson, E., Kearns, W.M., & Enzer, N. (1944). Effect of methyl testosterone on muscular performance and the central nervous system of older men. *Journal of Clinical Endocrinology & Metabolism*, **4**, 528-534.

Skakkebaek, N.E., Bancroft, J., Davidson, W., & Warner, P. (1981). Androgen replacement with oral testosterone undecanoate in hypogonadal men: A double blind controlled study. *Clinical Endocrinology*, **14**, 49-61.

Sourial, N., & Fenton, F. (1988). Testosterone treatment of an XXYY male presenting with aggression: A case report. *Canadian Journal of Psychiatry*, **33**, 846-850.

Steklis, H.D., Brammer, G.L., Raleigh, M.J., & McGuire, M.T. (1985). Serum testosterone, male dominance, and aggression in captive groups of vervet monkeys (Ceropithecus aethiops sabaeus). *Hormones and Behavior*, **19**, 154-163.

Stenn, P.G., Klaiber, E.L., Vogel, W., & Broverman, D.M. (1972). Testosterone effects upon photic stimulation of the electroencephalogram (EEG) and mental performance of humans. *Perceptual and Motor Skills*, **34**, 371-378.

Strauss, R.H., Ligget, M.T., & Lanese, R.R. (1985). Anabolic steroid use and perceived effects in ten weight-trained women athletes. *Journal of the American Medical Association*, **253**, 2871-2873.

Strauss, E.B., Sands, D.E., Robinson, A.M., Tindall, W.J., & Stevenson, W.A.H. (1952). Use of dehydroisoandrosterone in psychiatric treatment: A preliminary survey. *British Medical Journal*, **2**, 64-66.

Strauss, R.H., Wright, J.E., Finerman, G.A.M., & Catlin, D.H. (1983). Side effects of anabolic steroids in weight-trained men. *The Physician and Sportsmedicine*, **11**(2), 87-96.

Stumpf, W.E., & Sar, M. (1976). Steroid hormone target sites in the brain: The differential distribution of estrogen, progestin, androgen and glucocorticosteroid. *Journal of Steroid Biochemistry*, **7**, 1163-1170.

Susman, E.J., Inoff-Germain, G., Nottelmann, E.D., Loriaux, D.L., Cutler, G.B., & Chrousos, G.P. (1987). Hormones, emotional dispositions, and aggressive attributes in young adolescents. *Child Development*, **58**, 1114-1134.

Susman, E.J., Nottelmann, E.D., Inoff-Germain, G., Dorn, L.D., & Chrousos, G.P. (1987). Hormonal influences on aspects of psychological development during adolescence. *Journal of Adolescent Health Care*, **8**, 492-504.

Susman, E.J., Nottelmann, E.D., Inoff-Germain, G., Dorn, L.D., Cutler, G.B., Loriaux, D.L., & Chrousos, G.P. (1985). The relation of relative hormonal levels and physical development and social-emotional behavior in young adolescents. *Journal of Youth and Adolescence*, **14**(3), 245-264.

Svare, B.B. (1983). *Hormones and aggressive behavior*. New York: Plenum Press.

Svare, B.B. (1990). Anabolic steroids and behavior: A preclinical research prospectus. In G.C. Lin & L. Erinoff (Eds.), *Anabolic steroid abuse* (NIDA Research Monograph) (pp. 224-241). Rockville, MD: National Institute on Drug Abuse.

Tanaka, H., Yamamoto, K., Imamura, E., Yamauchi, M., Tanaka, M., Tamura, O., Inui, M., & Shindo, M. (1989). Relationship between plasma testosterone levels and psychological mood states or aptitudes in sportsmen. In *Proceedings of the First International Olympic Committee World Congress on Sports Science* (pp. 438-439). Colorado Springs, CO:

Table 10.8   Health Risk

Number of cycles	Definitely yes (%)	Probably yes (%)	Undecided (%)	Probably no (%)	Definitely no (%)	Total (%)
Sterility*						
1	50.0	30.0	17.5	2.5	0	100
2-4	29.9	32.0	23.7	10.3	4.1	100
≥ 5	24.4	4.9	19.5	12.2	39.0	100
Cancer*						
1	35.0	32.5	22.5	10.0	0	100
2-4	34.0	33.0	17.5	12.4	3.1	100
≥ 5	26.2	15.5	16.7	11.9	29.8	100
Heart attack*						
1	35.9	33.3	23.1	5.1	.6	100
2-4	37.5	33.3	15.6	10.4	3.1	100
≥ 5	22.9	16.9	18.1	10.9	31.3	100

Note. For sterility data, $\chi^2 = 35.82$; for cancer, $\chi^2 = 39.23$; for heart attack, $\chi^2 = 40.35$. Reprinted from Yesalis et al. (1989) by permission.

*$p < .0001$.

Table 10.9   Length of Cycles*

Number of cycles	<6 Weeks (%)	6-9 Weeks (%)	10-12 Weeks (%)	≥13 Weeks (%)	Total (%)
1	47.5	45.0	7.5	0	100
2-4	41.2	36.1	18.6	4.1	100
≥ 5	37.2	19.2	15.4	28.2	100

Note. $\chi^2 = 36.28$. Reprinted from Yesalis et al. (1989) by permission.

*$p < .0001$.

perceptions of peer use was a rationalization of use behavior on the part of the heavy users or the result of insider knowledge, the survey's approximate 7% use rate was applied to the total number of male seniors enrolled at each high school. This estimate of expected users at each school was then compared to the estimates given by the heavy users at each school. Almost without exception, the nonusers' estimate of peer anabolic steroid use was closer to the expected number calculated from the 7%-use rate than was the heavy users' estimate. Heavy users often estimated more than twice the expected number of users.

Table 10.10   Peer Use Perceptions*

How many students in your senior class do you think have ever used anabolic steroids?	Users (%)	Nonusers (%)
0	5.8	25.25
1-10	31.3	48.75
11-20	22.8	16.07
21-40	10.7	6.41
Over 40	29.5	3.52

Note. $\chi^2 = 341.1$. Reprinted from Yesalis et al. (1989) by permission.
*p < .0001.

Table 10.11   Peer Use Perceptions*

Number of cycles	0 (%)	1-10 (%)	11-20 (%)	21-40 (%)	40+ (%)	Total (%)
1	9.8	48.8	19.5	14.6	7.3	100
2-4	6.1	38.4	30.3	12.1	13.1	100
≥ 5	3.6	14.5	14.5	7.2	60.2	100

Note. $\chi^2 = 64.09$. Reprinted from Yesalis et al. (1989) by permission.
*p < .0001.

Finally, the variables listed in Tables 10.1 through 10.11 were cross-tabulated with age at time of first use of anabolic steroids. Not surprisingly, the perceptions of adolescents who initiated their anabolic steroid use before they were 16 years old were virtually identical in direction and magnitude to those of the heavy-user group described previously (data not displayed in tables). More importantly, only 9.5% of those students who reported initiating use at age 15 or younger reported having used only one cycle; 63% of these early starters reported having used more than five cycles.

Discussion

It is widely recognized that a drug's chemical structure alone does not predict its addictive effect. Both individual needs and expectations, for example, have a powerful effect on behavior following administration of

a drug (Hansen, Malotte, & Fielding, 1988). These psychological components are especially responsible for possible addictive outcomes. It is
interesting to note the similarities between attitudes of heavy anabolic
steroid users and those of other drug-dependent young people, for whom
the reinforcement strength of positive affective outcomes is a powerful
motivator to continue use. For an anabolic steroid user, feeling good about
oneself can result from increased self-esteem and positive peer admiration
that may be precipitated by improved appearance and performance. These
outcomes are strong reinforcers, as are the altered mood states that have
often been reported with higher levels of anabolic steroid use (e.g., increased self-confidence and feelings of euphoria and of well-being, sometimes to the point of true grandiosity, with hypomania or frank mania)
(Pope & Katz, 1988). Such psychological effects may be as strong in their
own right as the physical benefits of use.

The fact that steroid users, especially heavy users, perceive a greater
prevalence of use among peers than do nonusers suggests that, as the
intensity of use increases, users start to rationalize their actions and engage
in denial and projection as ways to justify their behavior (Semeonoff,
1976). This is similar to overestimation of peer use of other substances
found by Sherman et al. (1983) and Chassin et al. (1985). On the other
hand, the high estimates on the part of users may indicate a significant
underreporting of anabolic steroid use in this survey. Alternatively, the
heavy users may tend to associate to a greater extent with other anabolic
steroid users, a situation that may influence their perceptions of overall
use. This too parallels the actions of adolescents who use other drugs
(Kandel & Adler, 1982). Likewise, the dismissal of health risks, real or
perceived, is consistent with previous studies involving other adolescent
drug-use behaviors (Johnston et al., 1987). This hard-core group was
comprised primarily of adolescents who initiated their anabolic steroid
use at a younger age and who reported a greater number of episodes of
use. This is also consistent with outcome research that suggests that earlier
and heavier substance users are more likely to have problems associated
with use (Brunswick & Boyle, 1979; O'Donnell & Clayton, 1979; Robins &
Przybeck, 1985).

Several of the findings deserve additional comment. The use of injectable anabolic steroids indicates an increased level of commitment to this
drug behavior for two reasons: Few people other than addicts enjoy injections, and because insulin needles are not usually used for these injections,
users must obtain black-market, larger gauge needles (larger than 20
gauge). The use of injectable anabolic steroids can therefore lead to additional health problems associated with reusing or sharing needles, such
as AIDS and hepatitis. Sklarek, Montovani, and Erens (1984) have already
noted one case of AIDS in a bodybuilder who apparently shared needles
for anabolic steroid injection. More recently, two positive tests for human
immunodeficiency virus (HIV) among bodybuilders were attributed to

infected hypodermic needles used for injection of anabolic steroids (Scott & Scott, 1989; U.S. Olympic Committee, 1988). On the other hand, the orally active 17-α-alkylated anabolic steroids appear to have the greatest potential for direct health risk due to their hepatotoxicity and their ability to alter lipid states (Haupt & Rovere, 1984; Wilson, 1988; Wright, 1980; Yesalis, Wright, & Bahrke, 1989).

The fact that anabolic steroid users perceive their physical strength and health status to be better than that of their nonuser peers does not bode well for intervention strategies. Feeling good and looking good can be psychologically addicting and are obviously not incentives for terminating anabolic steroid use. We should note, however, that anabolic steroid users were also twice as likely as nonusers to report their health as fair or poor (11.2% vs. 5.8%, $p<.0001$). This is an inordinately high figure for this age group, 4 times above the national average (U.S. Department of Health and Human Services, 1987). It is not known whether this is a function of extremely high expectations of performance or of actual health problems; 70% of users who reported using anabolic steroids to treat injury reported their health as excellent. The group with the lowest health perceptions actually included those who reported using anabolic steroids because of peer pressure; 25% of these users reported their health as fair or poor. We must not overlook the potential for deleterious health effects among adolescent anabolic steroid users.

Conclusion

Data from the national survey suggest that the admitted use of anabolic steroids is currently much higher in the male adolescent population than was reported over a decade ago (Corder, Dezelsky, Toohey, & DiVito, 1975). It is particularly significant that approximately one-quarter of anabolic steroid users in the study reported behaviors, perceptions, and opinions that are consistent with psychological dependence, in terms of their unwillingness to stop use, their perceptions of risks and benefits of use, and their rationalization of use. Not surprisingly, this hard-core group is disproportionately comprised of heavy users and those who initiated use prior to age 16.

References

Adelson, J. (Ed.) (1980). *Handbook of adolescent psychology*. New York: Whale.

Bahrke, M., Yesalis, C., & Wright, J. (1990). Psychological and behavioral effects of endogenous testosterone levels and anabolic-androgenic steroids among males: A review. *Sports Medicine*, **10**, 303-337.

Brooks-Gunn, J., Petersen, A., Eichorn, D. (1985). The study of maturational timing effects in adolescence. *Journal of Youth and Adolescence*, **14**, 149-161.

Brower, K., Blow, F., Beresford, T., & Fuelling, C. (1989). Anabolic-androgenic steroid dependence. *Journal of Clinical Psychiatry*, **50**, 31-33.

Brunswick, A., & Boyle, J. (1979). Patterns of drug involvement: Developmental and secular influences on age of initiation. *Youth and Society*, **11**(2), 139-162.

Buckley, W., Yesalis, C., Friedl, K., Anderson, W., Streit, A., & Wright, J. (1988). Estimated prevalence of anabolic steroid use among male high school seniors. *Journal of the American Medical Association*, **260**, 3442-3445.

Chassin, L., Presson, C., & Sherman, S. (1985). Stepping backward in order to step forward: An acquisition-oriented approach to primary prevention. *Journal of Consulting and Clinical Psychology*, **53**(5), 612.

Corder, B., Dezelsky, T., Toohey, J., & DiVito, C. (1975). Trends in drug use behavior at ten central Arizona high schools. *Arizona Journal of Health, Physical Education, Recreation and Dance*, **18**(1), 10-11.

Crowley, T. (1988). Learning and unlearning drug abuse in the real world: Clinical treatment and public policy. In B. Ray (Ed.), *Learning factors in substance abuse* (NIDA Research Monograph No. 84, DHHS Publication No. ADM 88-1576). Rockville, MD: National Institute on Drug Abuse.

Hansen, W., Graham, J., Sobel, J., Shelton, D., Flay, B., & Johnson, C.A. (1987). The consistency of peer and parent influences in tobacco, alcohol and marijuana use among young adolescents. *Journal of Behavioral Medicine*, **10**, 559-579.

Hansen, W., Malotte, C., & Fielding, J. (1988). Evaluation of a tobacco and alcohol abuse prevention curriculum for adolescents. *Health Education Quarterly*, **15**(1), 93-114.

Haupt, H., & Rovere, G. (1984). Anabolic steroids: A review of the literature. *American Journal of Sports Medicine*, **12**(6), 469-484.

Hawkins, R., Lishner, D., Catalano, R., & Howard, M. (1986). Childhood predictors of adolescent substance abuse: Toward an empirically grounded theory. *Journal of Children in Contemporary Society*, **8**, 11-47.

Huba, G., Wingard, J., & Bentler, P. (1980). Framework for an interactive theory of drug use. In D. Lettieri, M. Sayers, & H. Person, (Eds.), *Theories on drug abuse* (NIDA Research Monograph No. 30, DHHS Publication No. ADM 80-967). Rockville, MD: National Institute on Drug Abuse.

Johnston, L., Bachman, J., O'Malley, P. (1991). *Monitoring the future: Continuing study of the lifestyles and values of youth*. Ann Arbor: University of Michigan Institute for Social Research.

Johnston, R., O'Malley, P., & Bachman, T. (1987). *National trends in drug use and related factors among American high school students and young adults, 1975-1986* (DHHS Publication No. ADM 87-1535). Rockville, MD: National Institute on Drug Abuse.

Kandel, D. (1978). *Longitudinal research of drug use: Empirical findings and methodological issues.* New York: Wiley.

Kandel, D., & Adler, I. (1982). Socialization into marijuana use among French adolescents: A cross-cultural comparison with the United States. *Journal of Health and Social Behavior*, **23**, 295-309.

Lerner, R. (1985). Adolescent maturational changes and psychosocial development: A dynamic interactional perspective. *Journal of Youth and Adolescents*, **14**, 355-372.

Newcomb, M., Maddahian, E., Skager, E., & Bentler, P. (1987). Substance abuse and psychosocial risk factors among teenagers: Associations with sex, age, ethnicity and type of school. *American Journal of Drug and Alcohol Abuse*, **13**, 413-433.

O'Donnell, J., & Clayton, R. (1979). Determinants of early marijuana use. In G. Beschner & A. Friedman (Eds.), *Youth drug abuse* (pp. 63-110). Lexington, MA: Lexington Books.

Pandina, R., Labouvie, E., & White, H. (1984). Potential contributions of the life span developmental approach to the study of adolescent alcohol and drug use: The Rutgers Health and Human Development Project, a working model. *Journal of Drug Issues*, **14**(2), 253-268.

Pope, H., & Katz, D. (1988). Affective and psychotic symptoms associated with anabolic steroid use. *American Journal of Psychiatry*, **145**(4), 487-490.

Robins, L., & Przybeck, T. (1985). Age of onset of drug use as a factor in drug and other disorders. In C. Jones & R. Baltjes (Eds.), *Etiology of drug abuse: Implications for prevention* (NIDA Research Monograph No. 56). Rockville, MD: National Institute on Drug Abuse.

Scott, J., & Scott, J. (1989). HIV infection with injections of anabolic steroids. *Journal of the American Medical Association*, **262**, 207-208.

Semeonoff, B. (1976). *Projective techniques.* London: Wiley.

Sherman, S., Presson, C., Chassin, L., Corty, E., & Olshavsky, R. (1983). The false consensus effect in estimates of smoking prevalence: Underlying mechanisms. *Personality and Social Psychology Bulletin*, **9**, 197-207.

Sklarek, H., Mantovani, R., & Evans, E. (1984). AIDS in a bodybuilder using anabolic steroids. *New England Journal of Medicine*, **311**(26), 1701.

Swisher, J., & Hu, T. (1983). Alternatives to drug abuse: Some are and some are not. In T. Glynn, C. Leukefeld, & J. Ludford (Eds.), *Preventing adolescent drug abuse* (NIDA Research Monograph No. 47). Rockville, MD: National Institute on Drug Abuse.

U.S. Department of Health and Human Services. (1987). *Health United States 1986 and prevention profile* (DHHS Publication No. PHS 87-1232). Washington, DC: U.S. Government Printing Office.

U.S. Olympic Committee. (1988, March). *Drug education news.* (Available from USOC, Colorado Springs, CO)

Wilson, J. (1988). Androgen abuse by athletes. *Endocrine Reviews,* **9**(2), 181-199.

Wright, J. (1978). *Anabolic steroids and sports.* Natick, MA: Sports Science Consultants.

Wright, J. (1980). Anabolic steroids and athletics. *Exercise and Sport Sciences Review,* **8**, 149-209.

Wright, J. (1982). *Anabolic steroids and sports: Volume II.* Natick, MA: Sports Science Consultants.

Yesalis, C.E., Vicary, J.R., Buckley, W.E., Streit, A.L., Katz, D.L., & Wright, J.E. (1990). Indications of psychological dependence among anabolic-androgenic steroid abusers. In G.C. Lin & L. Erinoff (Eds.), *Anabolic Steroid Abuse* (NIDA Research Monograph No. 102). Rockville, MD: National Institute on Drug Abuse.

Yesalis, C.E., Wright, J., & Bahrke, M. (1989). Epidemiologic and policy issues in the measurement of the long term health effects of anabolic-androgenic steroids. *Sports Medicine,* **8**(3), 29-138.

CHAPTER 11

Assessment and Treatment of Anabolic Steroid Withdrawal

Kirk J. Brower

The (Chargers) continued to offer Dianabol to the team as long as I was in San Diego. Civilian casualties were acceptable.

RON MIX
Former San Diego Charger
Member of the Football Hall of Fame
Sports Illustrated, October 19, 1987

Portions of this chapter are from Brower (1991); used by permission; see credits page for more information.

This chapter addresses two areas of concern for clinicians who treat anabolic steroid users. The first concern includes the identification and assessment of anabolic steroid users. For the purposes of the following discussion, *identification* refers to the detection of new cases, and *assessment* refers to the evaluation of known cases. Although the sports community has paid widespread attention to the identification of drug-using athletes via drug testing, little has been written about identifying anabolic steroid users in clinical practice via a careful search for the signs and symptoms associated with anabolic steroid use. Thus, this chapter will review the clinical manifestations of anabolic steroid use as might be evident during a history, physical examination, mental status examination, and laboratory examination. The second area of concern is the clinical management of anabolic steroid users who agree to stop using these drugs. Withdrawal from anabolic steroids may be problematic for some users, necessitating informed clinical care. Accordingly, this chapter will provide guidelines for the treatment of anabolic steroid withdrawal. Although the use of anabolic steroids has both sociocultural and biomedical implications, the major intent of this chapter is to place the problems associated with anabolic steroid use in a clinical context so they are subject to clinical interventions.

Identification and Assessment

Anabolic steroid users may present for treatment of the various side effects of their drug-taking without divulging their drug use. Surgeons may see bodybuilders who want treatment for gynecomastia (Aide, 1989), and dermatologists may see anabolic steroid users who want treatment for acne (Scott, 1989). Even when patients do admit to anabolic steroid use, a thorough assessment is indicated to guide the proper course of treatment (Brower, Catlin, Blow, Eliopulos, & Beresford, 1991).

Clinical identification, assessment, and treatment occur in the context of a confidential relationship. The clinician is not as interested in any punitive sanctions to which the patient may be subject, as in the health and well-being of the patient. Although some physicians have dual responsibilities to both sports organizations and patients, the emphasis here is on identification for clinical, not punitive, purposes. When the

This work was supported in part by NIAAA Grant 1P50AA07378-03.

clinical examination is conducted in the context of a confidential relationship, the patient can view the clinician as an ally rather than an adversary. This context should attenuate the tendency to deny drug use.

Epidemiologic studies indicate that young males who are recreational weight lifters, bodybuilders, or participants in sports that require strength or power are at highest risk for using anabolic steroids (Yesalis, Wright, & Lombardo, 1989). Thus, a high index of clinical suspicion for these patients is warranted, especially if the physical, mental status, or laboratory examinations reveal pertinent findings, as outlined in the following discussion.

History

The clinician may first ask the patient about his or her use of legal substances, such as alcohol and tobacco, then about nutrition and legal performance aids, such as protein supplements and amino acids. The clinician may then ask if the patient knows other people who have used or are using anabolic steroids. Finally, the clinician may ask if the patient has ever used anabolic steroids. If not, the patient should be asked if he or she has considered using anabolic steroids or if others have suggested it. The clinician and patient can then discuss the patient's reasons for not using or for considering use. Questions such as these can be useful for initiating a dialogue about anabolic steroids, for providing education, and for understanding both the personal goals of patients and the pressures they may experience to use anabolic steroids. The astute clinician will derive information from both the content of the patient's answers and the manner in which the patient responds. Nervousness, defensiveness, or evasiveness may be clues that the patient requires extra attention, even if anabolic steroid use is overtly denied. Corroborating history from a family member or a significant other can be extremely helpful in cases in which the patient appears to be in denial.

The *review of systems*, a standard part of history-taking when interviewing patients, should inquire about subjective complaints that have been associated with anabolic steroid use and withdrawal, such as headaches, dizziness, nausea, muscle spasms and aches, urinary frequency, and menstrual abnormalities (Haupt & Rovere, 1984). In addition, the clinician should look for psychiatric symptoms such as mood swings, depression, irritability, aggressiveness, increased or decreased energy level, disturbance in appetite, insomnia, dissatisfaction with one's physical appearance, and changes in libido (Brower, Catlin, et al., 1991). Finally, social dysfunction should be evaluated, such as arguments with or estrangement from family and friends, and decrements in performance on the job, at school, or on the playing field.

When patients do admit to using anabolic steroids, the clinician should determine the specific drugs used, source (licit or illicit), dosages, time of last use, duration of use, frequency of use, and routes of administration. A comprehensive inventory of other possibly used substances should be obtained, including opioids, aspirin, other nonsteroidal anti-inflammatory drugs, sedative-hypnotics, marijuana, alcohol, and tobacco (Wadler & Hainline, 1989). The clinician should determine use of substances that are taken to treat the side effects of anabolic steroids (e.g., estrogen blockers), to augment effects (e.g., human chorionic gonadotropin, growth hormone, erythropoietin, stimulants), and to mask use of anabolic steroids (e.g., diuretics, probenicid). Finally, the clinician should ascertain the degree of dependence on anabolic steroids by asking about efforts to stop or cut down, using more anabolic steroids than intended, continuing use despite adverse consequences, withdrawal symptoms, and tolerance (Brower, Blow, Young, & Hill, 1991) (see chapter 9).

Physical Examination

The following signs, arranged by system, may be associated with anabolic steroid use (Brower, Catlin, et al., 1991; Haupt & Rovere, 1984; Hickson, Ball, & Falduto, 1989; Kibble & Ross, 1987; Wilson, 1988). Some signs, such as high blood pressure, are not commonly seen, so they have little value for identification or screening but are important for assessment and monitoring of known cases. The absence of many signs, therefore, does not rule out anabolic steroid use, because some anabolic steroid users manifest relatively few side effects. Moreover, none of the following signs are specific for anabolic steroid use. Nevertheless, the presence of one or more of these signs in a high-risk patient should signal the possibility of anabolic steroid use.

Vital signs and physical dimensions—High blood pressure (Freed, Banks, Longson, & Burley, 1975; Lenders et al., 1988); marked, rapid weight gain with maintenance of, or increase in, lean body mass.

Skin—Acne; needle marks in large muscle groups (deltoids, gluteals); male pattern baldness; hirsutism in females; jaundice.

Head, eyes, ears, nose, and throat—Jaundiced eyes; deepened voice in females.

Chest—Gynecomastia in males; atrophied breasts in females.

Abdominal—Right upper quadrant tenderness; hepatomegaly (Ishak & Zimmerman, 1987).

Genitourinary—Testicular atrophy and prostatic hypertrophy in males; clitoral hypertrophy in females.

Musculoskeletal—Marked muscular hypertrophy; disproportionate development of the upper torso, especially the neck, shoulders, and chest.

Extremities—Edema.

Mental Status Exam

There is hardly a psychiatric symptom for which anabolic steroids have not been implicated in either causing or exacerbating (Bahrke, Yesalis, & Wright, 1990; Katz & Pope, 1990; Pope & Katz, 1988). The mental status exam is performed to obtain objective or observer-rated information about a patient's psychiatric condition. Although there may be scientific debate about the exact role of anabolic steroids in causing psychiatric disturbance, few would disagree that anabolic steroid users who exhibit one or more of the following signs require therapeutic attention. Therefore, the clinician should assess the following indicators of psychiatric disturbance.

Behavior—Psychomotor agitation or retardation, consistent with either manic or depressive disorders.

Mood—Euphoria; irritability; depression; marked anxiety.

Affect—Lability with abrupt shifts in moods.

Thought process—Slowed with depressive states; rapid or disorganized with manic states.

Thought content—Suicidal or homicidal thoughts; grandiose or persecutory thoughts that may progress to delusions.

Hallucinations

Laboratory Examination

Anabolic steroid users may show abnormalities of the following laboratory tests; thus, these tests should be ordered for those suspected of using anabolic steroids. Although urine testing for anabolic steroids should also be ordered (Brower, Catlin, et al., 1991), the following tests are usually more readily available with a faster turnaround time. In addition, the clinician can use laboratory abnormalities to alert the user of adverse consequences that require monitoring and intervention. Because normal reference values for the following tests may vary from laboratory to laboratory, clinicians should follow the normal reference range provided by their laboratories of use.

Liver function tests—Elevations in bilirubin, lactate dehydrogenase (LDH), alkaline phosphatase, aspartate amino transferase (AST, or SGOT), and alanine amino transferase (ALT, or SGPT—serum glutamic pyruvic transaminase) can be found (O'Connor, Skinner, Baldini, & Einstein, 1990). Serum levels of gamma-glutamyltransferase are not affected (Kiraly, 1988; Lenders et al., 1988). Elevations in ALT and AST can be due to intensive weight lifting even without anabolic steroid use and to intramuscular injections, due to the presence of these enzymes in skeletal muscle. Thus, liver-specific enzymes (e.g., the LDH isoenzyme) may be needed to rule out liver dysfunction (Haupt & Rovere, 1984).

Muscle enzymes—In addition to ALT and AST, elevations in creatine phosphokinase (CPK) have been observed in both steroid-using and nonusing weight lifters after a training session (Hakkinen & Alen, 1989). Anabolic steroid users, however, have even greater elevations than nonusers after exercising (Hakkinen & Alen, 1989), and they can have abnormal elevations in CPK before exercising (McKillop, Ballantyne, Borland, & Ballantyne, 1989). Serum creatinine may be elevated in both users and nonusers simply due to increased muscle bulk.

Cholesterol profile—Although total cholesterol may be elevated (O'Connor et al., 1990), the most consistent findings with 17-alkylated oral anabolic steroid administration are decreased levels of HDLC and increased levels of LDLC (Kiraly, 1988; Lenders et al., 1988; O'Connor et al., 1990). Triglycerides may also be elevated (O'Connor et al., 1990).

Hematocrit and hemoglobin—Due to the erythropoietic effect of anabolic steroids, the hematocrit and hemoglobin levels may be elevated relative to the patient's usual baseline level (Kiraly, 1988), although the hematocrit is rarely abnormally elevated (O'Connor et al., 1990). However, when athletes combine anabolic steroids with erythropoietin, as some endurance athletes have done, abnormal elevations are even more likely.

Endocrine tests of the pituitary-gonadal axis—Serum levels of luteinizing hormone (LH) and follicular-stimulating hormone (FSH) are reduced in response to the feedback inhibition of exogenously administered anabolic steroids on the hypothalamus and pituitary gland (Alen & Rahkila, 1988). Serum testosterone levels may be increased with the use of testosterone esters (that are metabolized to testosterone) but decreased with the exclusive use of other anabolic steroids or following cessation of anabolic steroid use (Alen, Reinila, & Vihko, 1985). Similarly, serum estradiol levels may be either increased or decreased, depending on the use of testosterone esters (which are also metabolized to estradiol) and depending on whether the user is on a cycle or between cycles of use.

Semen analysis—Sperm count and motility may be decreased, and sperm morphology may be abnormal (Knuth, Maniera, & Nieschlag, 1989).

Glucose tolerance test—Although fasting serum glucose levels are not affected, one study revealed that anabolic steroid users had diminished 2-hr glucose tolerance tests when compared to controls (Cohen & Hickman, 1987). Nevertheless, none of the anabolic steroid users had abnormal tests indicative of diabetes. Thus, the value of the glucose tolerance test as a marker of anabolic steroid use is unproven.

Cardiac function tests—There are a few case reports in the medical literature of myocardial infarction (MI) in anabolic steroid users. Although the value of an electrocardiogram (EKG) to screen for occult MIs in anabolic steroid users is unknown, a baseline EKG is recommended for known or suspected users. Electrocardiographic evidence of left ventricular hypertrophy (LVH) is likely in bodybuilders and strength athletes who use anabolic steroids (Urhausen, Holpes, & Kindermann, 1989), although this finding may be seen in nonusing strength athletes as well (Alpert, Pape, Ward, & Rippe, 1989). Nevertheless, some (Urhausen, Holpes, & Kindermann, 1989), but not all (Zuliani et al., 1988) studies reveal that the LVH in anabolic steroid users is associated with impaired diastolic function, and so a clinician should consider an echocardiogram for a patient with EKG evidence of LVH.

Treatment of Withdrawal

The clinical management of withdrawal from high-dose, illicit anabolic steroid use is completely unstudied. At the time of this writing, there were no publications of controlled (or even uncontrolled) studies that evaluated treatment protocols for withdrawal from anabolic steroids. Indeed, among the few case reports of anabolic steroid dependence in the literature (Brower, Blow, Beresford, & Fuelling, 1989; Hays, Littleton, & Stillner, 1990; Tennant, Black, & Voy, 1988), the treatment outcomes were invariably characterized by "lost to follow-up." As such, the following approaches are based on limited numbers of patients seen in the author's clinical practice and on personal communications with other practicing physicians who treat illicit steroid users.

Symptoms of withdrawal from anabolic steroids include depressed mood, fatigue, muscle and joint pain, restlessness, anorexia, insomnia, decreased libido, headache, and the desire to take more steroids (craving) (Brower, Blow, et al., 1991; Brower, Eliopulos, Blow, Catlin, & Beresford, 1990; Kashkin & Kleber, 1989; see also Table 9.2, p. 201). The most life-threatening complication of withdrawal from anabolic steroids that has been reported to date is suicidal depression (Brower, Blow, Eliopulos, & Beresford, 1989; Elofson & Elofson, 1990). Obviously, therefore, withdrawal symptoms may be severe enough to warrant treatment. Some authors hypothesize that withdrawal from anabolic steroids is biphasic in nature, with an initial phase marked by hyperadrenergic symptoms resembling opioid withdrawal and a later phase marked predominantly by depressive symptoms and craving (Kashkin & Kleber, 1989). Unfortunately, the validity and durations of these phases have not been adequately studied or described. Roughly estimated, Phase 1 begins within 1 to 2 days of cessation of use and lasts for about 1 week; Phase 2 may begin in the 1st week and can last for several months. If this theory is borne out by future research, treatment may need to be accordingly biphasic.

The goals of treatment are

- to alleviate distressing withdrawal symptoms and prevent complications,
- to facilitate and initiate abstinence from illicit anabolic steroids,
- to prevent relapse to further use of anabolic steroids, and
- to restore the functioning of the hypothalamic-pituitary-gonadal (HPG) axis.

Therapeutic Alternatives

The treatment of withdrawal from anabolic steroids may be thought of as detoxification. As with other drugs of abuse, steroid detoxification consists of supportive therapy with or without pharmacotherapy (see Table 11.1). (Steroid abusers may be concomitantly dependent on other substances, such as alcohol, for which other specific detoxification measures are indicated. Assessment, therefore, needs to include a history of the full range of addictive substance use.)

Table 11.1   Treatment Alternatives for Anabolic Steroid Withdrawal

I. Supportive therapy
II. Pharmacotherapy
   A. For hypothalamic-pituitary-gonadal dysfunction
      1. Testosterone esters
      2. Human chorionic gonadotropin (HCG)
      3. Antiestrogens (clomiphene, tamoxifen)
      4. Short-acting LHRH agonists
   B. For symptomatic relief and/or treatment of coexisting disorders
      1. Antidepressants
      2. Clonidine
      3. Nonsteroidal anti-inflammatory drugs (NSAIDs)
      4. Tranquilizers
         a. Neuroleptics (with or without lithium)
         b. Benzodiazepines
         c. Antihistamines (diphenhydramine, hydroxyzine)

Note. Please see text for specific recommendations. Reprinted from Brower (1991) by permission.

Supportive Therapy

Supportive therapy refers to psychological measures such as reassurance, education, and counseling. Patients are most reassured when the clinician is nonjudgmental, understanding, and knowledgeable about anabolic steroids and withdrawal. The need to establish a therapeutic alliance with the patient cannot be overstated. For both pharmacological and psychological reasons, a patient may initially be aggressive and combative and may thus perceive the clinician as an opponent (B. Goldman, personal communication, 1990). If the clinician is also an athlete, he or she may use this to advantage for establishing rapport. If not, then the patient needs other evidence that the clinician understands his or her condition from both a medical and nonmedical perspective. More specifically, the clinician needs to understand the patient's point of view, because patients perceive their reasons for taking anabolic steroids as good ones. Almost invariably, the illicit steroid user is extremely invested in his or her physical attributes and body image. When the clinician understands these and other reasons for drug-taking, he or she can counsel the patient about finding acceptable alternatives.

Acceptable alternatives for a bodybuilder, for example, may include nutritional counseling and consultation with an exercise physiologist or other fitness expert, who can both assist the patient with setting realistic training goals and provide safe regimens to achieve them. Although these substitutes probably will not provide the same physical gains that anabolic steroids can, the psychological benefits of substitutes can be powerful both for engaging patients in treatment and for preventing relapse. Moreover, the selection of appropriate substitutes conveys to patients that their needs have been understood.

Clinicians should educate patients about what they may experience during withdrawal, including depressed mood. By anticipating possible symptoms, the patient is reassured by the clinician's knowledge if such symptoms should occur. If symptoms have already occurred, the patient is reassured by the explanation that these are withdrawal symptoms rather than something intrinsically wrong with the patient or his or her character.

Although the clinician neither condones nor facilitates the drug-taking, persuasion to discontinue anabolic steroids should be based on health concerns rather than moralistic ones. In this regard, education about the health effects of anabolic steroids is important. The clinician can reinforce and personalize education by giving feedback to the patient about his or her own abnormal clinical findings or laboratory values. During abstinence, the clinician and patient can follow reversible abnormalities—such as testicular atrophy or abnormal cholesterol profiles—that provide concrete and reassuring evidence of improvement. Steroid users invariably believe that these drugs improve physical attributes in a variety of ways. Although a minority of experts still dispute the efficacy of anabolic steroids for these uses (Wilson, 1988), attempts to dissuade steroid users are fruitless and serve no clinical purpose. Rather, the clinician should agree that these are very potent drugs, then raise further concerns about their potential for causing adverse consequences.

Supportive therapy is always indicated during withdrawal, because the risks of suicidal depression and relapse are especially high during this period (Brower, Blow, Eliopulos, & Beresford, 1989; Elofson & Elofson, 1990). Clinicians should ask patients if they feel depressed and if they have ever felt so depressed that they thought about killing themselves. Patients should be encouraged to discuss these feelings if they occur. When the patient is suicidal, consultation with a psychiatrist is advisable.

Pharmacotherapy

Pharmacotherapy is considered to be adjunctive to supportive therapy. Pharmacotherapy is indicated when the clinical symptoms, with or without laboratory evidence of HPG dysfunction, are persistently severe. *Persistently severe* is not precisely defined, because each patient's treatment plan should be decided individually. As long as the patient can tolerate the withdrawal symptoms and responds to supportive therapy, however, watchful waiting is the prudent strategy. Pharmacotherapy is contraindicated when the patient cannot make a commitment to abstinence, because the physician may then be facilitating drug-taking behavior as well as the likelihood of an adverse drug interaction between the physician's prescribed drug and the patient's illicit drugs. Contraindications and precautions for specific agents are noted as follows.

Pharmacotherapy can be divided into two major types: drugs that are targeted specifically at the HPG axis to restore HPG functioning, and drugs that are targeted at specific withdrawal symptoms to provide symptomatic relief, regardless of HPG axis functioning. The first group includes testosterone esters, human chorionic gonadotropin (HCG), estrogen blockers such as clomiphene, and synthetic forms of gonadotropin-releasing hormone such as leuprolide. The second group includes antidepressants, nonnarcotic analgesics, clonidine, and tranquilizers.

Pharmacotherapy for HPG Axis Functioning

The prolonged use of high-dose anabolic steroids results in hypogonadotropic hypogonadism (Alen & Rahkila, 1988; Jarow & Lipshultz, 1990). Before initiating pharmacotherapy of this type, therefore, a physician should determine baseline levels of serum testosterone, estradiol, leuteinizing hormone (LH), and follicular stimulating hormone. Sperm counts may also be useful in some cases. Pharmacotherapy for HPG axis functioning is indicated only in the presence of clinically significant symptoms and abnormalities of these laboratory parameters. Because of the dearth of clinical experience with these drugs for the treatment of anabolic steroid withdrawal, combined in some cases (i.e., clomiphene and leuprolide) with the lack of approval by the Food and Drug Administration (FDA) for treating hypogonadotropic hypogonadism, these approaches are recommended mainly as an impetus for designing research protocols. Furthermore, these pharmacotherapies are based on the rationale of restoring HPG axis functioning in men. Case descriptions of anabolic steroid withdrawal in women are lacking, although some agents are used in women to treat infertility (HCG, clomiphene, gonadorelin), breast cancer (tamoxifen), and endometriosis (nafarelin). In addition, notwithstanding the use of HCG to treat boys with cryptorchidism and hypogonadotropic hypogonadism, and the use of testosterone esters to treat boys with hypogonadism, micropenis, and delayed puberty, these agents are infrequently used in children. Thus, endocrine pharmacotherapy for female and pediatric steroid users must be carefully weighed. Nonspecialists in endocrinology should consult with gynecologic and pediatric endocrinologists before initiating endocrine therapies in women and children, respectively. Consultation with an endocrinologist is also advisable when treating adult males.

Testosterone Esters.   A common approach to detoxification for other drugs of abuse is to substitute a long-acting drug with cross-tolerance and then taper the substituted drug. For example, chlordiazepoxide, a long-acting benezodiazepine with cross-tolerance to ethanol, is a drug of choice for alcohol detoxification. Likewise, high therapeutic doses of a testosterone ester can be substituted for the illicit steroid regimen and then tapered at 1- to 2-week intervals. For example, an initial injection of 200 to 400 mg of testosterone enanthate can be decreased by 50 to 100 mg every 1 to 2 weeks. A single injection of testosterone enanthate (200 mg) has been reported to alleviate withdrawal symptoms in 1 to 2 days in patients whose serum testosterone levels are low (D. Coleman, personal communication, 1990).

Inasmuch as withdrawal symptoms are correlated with persistent depression of the HPG axis, then a tapering course of testosterone enanthate shares an analogous rationale to a tapering course of corticosteroids following chronic use of those drugs. Although theoretically plausible, this approach presents a number of difficulties. First, prescription of an abused substance to a substance abuser can be problematic unless closely supervised. Thus, the medical administration of anabolic steroids for detoxification should occur only in the physician's office or clinic, and self-administration of take-home prescriptions should be avoided.

Unfortunately, steroid abusers might readily agree to medically administered injections as a means to bolster their illicit, self-administered steroid regimens. In these cases, urine testing for the illicit use of anabolic steroids may prove valuable. Second, the initial dose for taper can be

difficult to determine, because illicit steroid users typically consume between 10 to 100 times the therapeutic dosage (Wilson, 1988), and their
regimens often include both falsely labeled and veterinary preparations
for which the human dose is incalculable. Thus, the physician may need to
titrate the medically administered dose against the severity of withdrawal
symptoms on an empirical basis. Third, the substitution of testosterone
esters may provide symptomatic relief but actually prolong the recovery
time of the HPG axis by continuing to suppress hypothalamic-pituitary
function. Thus, other medication for symptomatic relief may be preferable.

Human Chorionic Gonadotropin.   During withdrawal, steroid abusers have abnormally low serum testosterone and LH values (Alen, Reinila, & Vihko, 1985), and they resemble prepubertal boys in their responses
to HCG (Martikainen, Alen, Rahkila, & Vihko, 1986). During withdrawal,
a single dose of 50 IU/kg can double serum testosterone levels at 3 to 4
days after HCG administration (Martikainen et al., 1986). For treatment
of steroid withdrawal, the dosage of HCG need not exceed that recommended by the manufacturer for treatment of male hypogonadism. Therapy can be continued for 4 to 6 weeks or until serum LH values return to
normal. Physicians need to be aware that HCG is sold illicitly to stimulate
endogenous testosterone production and to prevent testicular atrophy in
steroid users; thus, prescription-seeking for HCG can occur for diversion
to the black market.

Clomiphene.   Estradiol levels can increase during illicit androgen administration due to peripheral aromatization. Indeed, male steroid abusers
not uncommonly self-administer antiestrogenic agents (such as tamoxifen
or clomiphene) to prevent bothersome, feminizing side effects such as
gynecomastia (Friedl & Yesalis, 1989). Once again, therefore, the physician
must be alert to prescription-seeking for illegal diversion. As with exogenous anabolic steroids, high estradiol levels may suppress gonadotropin
secretion via feedback inhibition at the hypothalamic-pituitary level. Clomiphene may increase secretion of gonadotropins by preventing this feedback inhibition. Although estradiol levels can be expected to return to
physiological values within 3 weeks of discontinued use of androgens,
serum testosterone may take 12 or more weeks to return to normal (Alen
et al., 1985). Clomiphene may be useful not only when serum estradiol
levels are high but also when serum estradiol has returned to normal
while the serum testosterone level remains depressed. During this latter
hormonal configuration, clomiphene may result both in a more favorable
ratio of testosterone-to-estradiol activity and in diminished feedback inhibition of LH secretion. One approach is to prescribe 50 mg twice daily for
10 to 14 days, which can be repeated according to symptomatic response
and serial measures of serum testosterone and LH (D. Coleman, personal
communication, 1990). However, clomiphene is FDA-approved only for

the treatment of female infertility. Whether tamoxifen (approved only for the treatment of metastatic breast cancer in women) might have any advantages over clomiphene for the treatment of anabolic steroid withdrawal is unknown.

Leuprolide. Leuprolide acetate is a synthetic analog of leuteinizing hormone–releasing hormone (LHRH) that is FDA-approved only for the treatment of prostate cancer. Daily administration of LHRH (1 mg subcutaneously) for 1 week leads to an increase in serum LH and testosterone levels, whereas daily administration for more than 1 week leads to a decrease in these levels. Theoretically, then, brief treatment with a short-acting LHRH analog may have a place in the pharmacological armamentarium for treating anabolic steroid withdrawal. However, in the absence of further research, LHRH for the treatment of anabolic steroid withdrawal cannot be recommended because clinical experience with this approach is exceedingly sparse.

Other Forms of Synthetic LHRH. Synthetic LHRH is currently available in three other forms in addition to leuprolide. The goserelin acetate implant is a long-acting LHRH analog that is indicated to treat prostate cancer. Because it lasts for 28 days, it leads to a decrease in LH and testosterone, and thus is contraindicated in the treatment of anabolic steroid withdrawal. Nafarelin nasal spray is a short-acting LHRH analog that is approved for the treatment of endometriosis. Like leuprolide, it leads to initial stimulation of LH and FSH, followed by a decrease. Gonadorelin acetate is a synthetic form of LHRH that is administered to women by pulsatile intravenous injection to treat infertility caused by primary hypothalamic amenorrhea. Because a physiologic dose of gonadorelin acetate is delivered into the vein by a special pump device every 90 minutes, approximating the pulsatile rate of the natural hormone, LH is stimulated for the duration of the treatment period.

Pharmacotherapy for Symptomatic Relief

This group includes antidepressants, clonidine, nonnarcotic analgesics, and tranquilizers.

Antidepressants. Because the majority of withdrawal symptoms are depressive in nature, antidepressant treatment may be indicated. One uncontrolled study revealed that 12% of steroid users suffered from a "clinical" or major depression during the first 3 months after stopping the use of anabolic steroids (Pope & Katz, 1988). Even in the absence of a clinical or major depression, however, antidepressants may prove effective in treating anabolic steroid withdrawal and in diminishing craving, as they have in the treatment of cocaine withdrawal (Gawin et al., 1989). Nevertheless, the indication for antidepressant therapy is bolstered when a coexisting reason for its use exists, such as major depression, panic disorder, obsessive-compulsive disorder, cocaine dependence, migraine headaches, or chronic pain. Unlike the agents previously discussed (e.g., testosterone, HCG, clomiphene), antidepressants are not likely to be abused or diverted for illicit sales.

The therapeutic action of the antidepressants is generally attributed to their effects on various neurotransmitter systems, particularly serotonergic and noradrenergic systems. As science begins to better understand the interactions of anabolic steroids with these neurotransmitter systems, we may be able to select antidepressants based on their relative specificities for certain neurotransmitters. At this time, however, there is no reason to expect that any particular antidepressant is superior to any other for the treatment of steroid withdrawal. Antidepressants do differ in terms of their side-effect profiles and in the availability of established therapeutic blood levels. Moreover, certain disorders that may coexist (as cited previously) have responded differentially to specific antidepressants. These differences can influence the selection of a particular agent for a particular patient.

Some antidepressants have considerable overdose potential and may potentiate the adverse cardiac effects reported in steroid users. The physician must carefully assess the potentials for cardiotoxicity and suicide, therefore, before starting antidepressants. Patients should have baseline and serial EKGs, orthostatic pulse and blood pressure measurements, and close monitoring of any cardiac symptoms. Antidepressants with high anticholinergic activity should either be avoided or used with caution in patients with steroid-induced (or steroid-exacerbated) prostatic hypertrophy, in order to prevent urinary retention.

The same doses that are recommended for the treatment of depression are recommended for anabolic steroid withdrawal. In general, the physician gradually raises the dose until either symptomatic relief is obtained or bothersome side effects are experienced. Unfortunately, optimal effects may not take place until 2 to 6 weeks after adequate dosing has been achieved. Thus, patience on the part of both the physician and patient is required to ensure an adequate trial of therapy. In the interim, other treatment measures may be needed. The duration of therapy will depend on the responsiveness of symptoms, the presence of coexisting disorders, and the potential for relapse. For treatment of major depression, therapy is usually continued for 6 to 12 months.

Clonidine.   One case report suggested that the initial stage of anabolic steroid withdrawal is marked by hyperadrenergic symptoms resembling opioid withdrawal (Tennant et al., 1988). These symptoms were precipitated by a naloxone challenge and included nausea, headache, diaphoresis, piloerection, chills, dizziness, and increased pulse and blood pressure. Clonidine, which ameliorates opioid withdrawal, was noted to suppress these symptoms as well. Although dosage was not specified, 0.1 mg of clonidine every 4 to 6 hours by mouth is generally given on the 1st day of treatment for opioid withdrawal, is increased daily as needed by 0.1 to 0.2 mg to a maximum of 1.2 mg/day, and is then gradually tapered by 0.1 to 0.2 mg/day (Guthrie, 1990). Major side effects are hypotension and sedation, which require careful monitoring and possible adjustment of dosage. Because sedation may be poorly tolerated by patients who are already feeling depressed and fatigued, and who generally strive to feel strong at all costs, clonidine is not recommended unless there is clear evidence of opioidlike withdrawal symptoms. Indeed, the presence of such symptoms has not been well documented during anabolic steroid withdrawal, and the use of opioid withdrawal rating scales may be useful in this regard for both clinical and research purposes (Handelsman et al., 1987).

Analgesics.   Steroid users maintain that anabolic steroids decrease their recovery time between workouts, allowing them to train for longer hours and more frequently without experiencing fatigue or pain. The added muscle bulk, however, places extra stress on tendons and ligaments that can lead to injury or inflammation. During withdrawal, patients commonly experience muscle and joint pains that partly reflect the extreme, exertional effects of intensive training but without the attenuation of pain that anabolic steroids might possibly provide. Headaches are also frequently reported. Whether the musculoskeletal pains and headaches bear any resemblance to the discomforts of opioid withdrawal is unknown. In either case, nonsteroidal anti-inflammatory drugs (NSAIDs), such as ibuprofen or naproxen, may represent the analgesic drugs of choice for the headaches and musculoskeletal pains of anabolic steroid withdrawal. NSAIDS are not addictive (an important consideration in someone who is abusing anabolic steroids and perhaps other drugs), provide effective analgesia, and counter the inflammation resulting from overstressed ligaments and tendons.

Certain side effects of the NSAIDs, albeit rare (less than 3% of patients), are of particular concern in steroid abusers. For example, NSAIDs can cause elevations in liver function tests, which may already be elevated due to the patient's anabolic steroid use. Thus, monitoring of liver function tests is important. These agents may also result in edema and fluid retention, as can anabolic steroids; this is especially important if cardiac function has been affected by the use of anabolic steroids. In addition, NSAIDs have been associated with psychiatric symptoms such as nervousness, depression, and emotional lability. The main disadvantage of these agents, therefore, is their potential to either mask or retard improvement of the hepatic, cardiovascular, or central nervous system effects of the anabolic steroids. In actual practice, however, the likelihood of this occurring is probably small. Nevertheless, the physician must be alert to the possibility of these side effects when initiating and monitoring the course of treatment. Finally, these agents are contraindicated in the presence of angioedema, a condition for which anabolic steroids are legitimately prescribed.

Tranquilizers.   Major tranquilizers, or neuroleptics, are indicated in the presence of psychotic symptoms or acute mania. Physicians should also consider these drugs for treating marked irritability, aggressiveness, or agitation. As with corticosteroid-induced psychosis or mania, the addition of lithium may be considered. Long-term treatment with neuroleptics will probably be unwarranted in most cases, and these drugs can be tapered over a period of days to weeks after symptoms have subsided. Although minor tranquilizers, of which benzodiazepines are the drugs of choice, can alleviate short-term anxiety symptoms associated with withdrawal, the physician must carefully weigh their potential for paradoxically causing aggressiveness, although rare, in a patient who may already exhibit signs of aggressiveness. Nevertheless, some authors have suggested that benzodiazepines may be useful in the treatment of anabolic steroid withdrawal that is characterized by hyperadrenergic symptoms (Rosse & Deutsch, 1990). The antihistamines hydroxyzine and diphenhydramine have also been used as antianxiety agents and should be considered as alternatives to the benzodiazepines, although their anticholinergic side effects may preclude their use in the presence of prostatic hypertrophy.

Indications for Hospitalization

When the patient is suicidal, hospitalization may be needed. Other patients may manifest irritability and hostility during the initial withdrawal period. If the patient has been violent or presents a danger to others, then hospitalization is usually required. A third indication for hospitalization occurs when the patient has been unable to initiate abstinence as an outpatient.

Preferred Approach

In the absence of studies demonstrating the efficacy of pharmacotherapies, the preferred approach is rapid discontinuation of anabolic steroids, supportive therapy, and watchful waiting. If symptoms are prolonged or severe, then pharmacotherapy and/or hospitalization may be needed. All patients require an evaluation for suicidal thoughts.

In terms of pharmacotherapy directed at the HPG axis, HCG is considered the most promising approach for the following reasons. First, there is research evidence that steroid abusers during withdrawal respond to

HCG with increased testosterone levels (Martikainen et al., 1986). Second, the injections can be administered in the physician's office, thereby maintaining periodic contact with the patient for monitoring and support as well as preventing illegal diversion of prescription drugs. Third, HCG has FDA approval in the treatment of hypogonadotropic hypogonadism, a condition that characterizes withdrawal from anabolic steroids. Fourth, HCG stimulates the testes and should not lead to further suppression of the HPG axis, as might occur with the administration of testosterone esters.

In terms of pharmacotherapy for symptomatic relief, each of the agents deserves consideration depending upon which symptoms dominate the clinical picture. However, antidepressants and NSAIDs will likely be the most commonly used agents, because depressive symptoms, craving, and musculoskeletal pains are frequently reported and can easily lead to resumed use of anabolic steroids.

Pros and Cons of Treatment

Supportive therapy is necessary but requires a psychological orientation and can be time-intensive. Patients may require referrals to clinicians who provide this type of care if the treating physician is not so inclined. Pharmacotherapy offers the hope of more rapid relief of symptoms and restoration of HPG functioning. It is essential for the treatment of coexisting diagnoses such as major depression or psychosis but is considered adjunctive in the treatment of anabolic steroid withdrawal. Unfortunately, pharmacotherapy is completely unstudied for the treatment of anabolic steroid withdrawal, and each of the agents has its own side effects that the physician must consider. Moreover, patients may abuse some of the drugs given to them or divert them for illicit sales.

Although providing supportive therapy and pharmacological relief of symptoms may facilitate both initial abstinence and trust in the physician, the treatment of withdrawal symptoms (detoxification) is only the first step in managing steroid dependence. Patients may require rehabilitation to rebuild their lives without the use of anabolic steroids and other drugs (Brower, 1989). Further clinical research is needed to determine the optimal combinations of treatment for anabolic-androgenic steroid withdrawal and dependence.

Conclusions

Knowledge of the clinical manifestations of anabolic steroid use will help clinicians identify and assess anabolic steroid users. The highest risk patients are young males who lift weights for the purposes of enhancing either athletic performance or physical appearance. Among users, clinicians should ascertain signs and symptoms of dependence, because specialized treatment may be indicated. Although optimal treatment strategies must await further research, attention to both pharmacological and psychosocial factors is crucial in steroid withdrawal treatment, as with the treatment of other substance problems.

References

Aide, A.E. (1989). Surgical treatment of gynecomastia in the body builder. *Plastic and Reconstructive Surgery*, **83**, 61-66.

Alen, M., & Rahkila, P. (1988). Anabolic-androgenic steroid effects on endocrinology and lipid metabolism in athletes. *Sports Medicine*, **6**, 327-332.

Alen, M., Reinila, M., & Vihko, R. (1985). Response of serum hormones to androgen administration in power athletes. *Medicine and Science in Sports and Exercise*, **17**, 354-359.

Alpert, J.S., Pape, L.A., Ward, A., & Rippe, J.M. (1989). Athletic heart syndrome. *The Physician and Sportsmedicine*, **17**(7), 103-107.

Bahrke, M., Yesalis, C., & Wright, J. (1990). Psychological and behavioral effects of endogenous testosterone and anabolic-androgenic steroids among males: A review. *Sports Medicine*, **10**, 303-337.

Brower, K.J. (1989). Rehabilitation for anabolic-androgenic steroid dependence. *Clinical Sports Medicine*, **1**, 171-181.

Brower, K.J. (1991). Withdrawal from anabolic steroids. In C.W. Bardin (Ed.), *Current therapy in endocrinology and metabolism* (4th ed.) (pp. 259-264). Philadelphia: B.C. Decker.

Brower, K.J., Blow, F.C., Beresford, T.P., & Fuelling, C. (1989). Anabolic-androgenic steroid dependence. *Journal of Clinical Psychiatry*, **50**, 31-33.

Brower, K.J., Blow, F.C., Eliopulos, G.A., & Beresford, T.P. (1989). Anabolic-androgenic steroids and suicide [Letter to the editor]. *American Journal of Psychiatry*, **146**, 1075.

Brower, K.J., Blow, F.C., Young, J.A., & Hill, E.M. (1991). Symptoms and correlates of anabolic-androgenic steroid dependence. *British Journal of Addiction*, **86**, 759-768.

Brower, K.J., Catlin, D.H., Blow, F.C., Eliopulos, G.A., & Beresford, T.P. (1991). Clinical assessment and urine testing for anabolic-androgenic steroid abuse and dependence. *American Journal of Drug and Alcohol Abuse*, **17**, 161-171.

Brower, K.J., Eliopulos, G.A., Blow, F.C., Catlin, D.H., & Beresford, T.P. (1990). Evidence for physical and psychological dependence on anabolic androgenic steroids in eight weight lifters. *American Journal of Psychiatry*, **147**, 510-512.

Cohen, J.C., & Hickman, R. (1987). Insulin resistance and diminished glucose tolerance in powerlifters ingesting anabolic steroids. *Journal of Clinical Endocrinology and Metabolism*, **64**, 960-963.

Elofson, G., & Elofson, S. (1990). Steroids claimed our son's life. *The Physician and Sportsmedicine*, **18**, 15-16.

Freed, D.L., Banks, A.J., Longson, D., & Burley, D.M. (1975). Anabolic steroids in athletics: Crossover double-blind trial on weightlifters. *British Medical Journal*, **2**, 471-473.

Friedl, K.E., & Yesalis, C.E. (1989). Self-treatment of gynecomastia in bodybuilders who use anabolic steroids. *The Physician and Sportsmedicine*, **17**, 67-79.

Gawin, F.H., Kleber, H.D., Byck, R., Rounsaville, B.J., Kosten, T.R., Jatlow, P.I., & Morgan, C. (1989). Desipramine facilitation of initial cocaine abstinence. *Archives of General Psychiatry*, **46**, 117-121.

Guthrie, S. (1990). The pharmacotherapy of heroin withdrawal. *The Michigan Drug Letter*, **9**(8), 1-6.

Hakkinen, K., & Alen, M. (1989). Training volume, androgen use and serum creatine kinase activity. *British Journal of Sports Medicine*, **23**, 188-189.

Handelsman, L., Cochrane, K.J., Aronson, M.J., Ness, R., Rubinstein, K.J., & Kanof, P.D. (1987). Two new rating scales for opiate withdrawal. *American Journal of Drug and Alcohol Abuse*, **13**, 293-308.

Haupt, H.A., & Rovere, G.D. (1984). Anabolic steroids: A review of the literature. *American Journal of Sports Medicine*, **12**, 469-484.

Hays, L.R., Littleton, S., & Stillner, V. (1990). Anabolic steroid dependence [Letter to the editor]. *American Journal of Psychiatry*, **147**, 122.

Hickson, R.C., Ball, K.L., & Falduto, M.T. (1989). Adverse effects of anabolic steroids. *Medical Toxicology and Adverse Drug Experience*, **4**, 254-271.

Ishak, K.G., & Zimmerman, H.J. (1987). Hepatotoxic effects of the anabolic/androgenic steroids. *Seminars in Liver Disease*, **7**, 230-236.

Jarow, J.P., & Lipshultz, L.I. (1990). Anabolic steroid-induced hypogonadotropic hypogonadism. *American Journal of Sports Medicine*, **18**, 429-431.

Kashkin, K.B., & Kleber, H.D. (1989). Hooked on hormones? An anabolic steroid addiction hypothesis. *Journal of the American Medical Association*, **262**, 3166-3170.

Katz, D.L., & Pope, H.G., Jr. (1990). Anabolic-androgenic steroid-induced mental status changes. *National Institute on Drug Abuse Research Monograph Series*, **102**, 215-223.

Kibble, M.W., & Ross, M.B. (1987). Adverse effects of anabolic steroids in athletes. *Clinical Pharmacy*, **6**, 686-692.

Kiraly, C.L. (1988). Androgenic-anabolic steroid effects on serum and skin surface lipids, on red cells, and on liver enzymes. *International Journal of Sports Medicine*, **9**, 249-252.

Knuth, U.A., Maniera, H., & Nieschlag, E. (1989). Anabolic steroids and semen parameters in bodybuilders. *Fertility and Sterility*, **52**, 1041-1047.

Lenders, J.W.M., Demacker, P.N.M., Vos, J.A., Jansen, P.L.M., Hoitsma, A.J., van't Lar, A., & Thien, T. (1988). Deleterious effects of anabolic steroids on serum lipoproteins, blood pressure, and liver function in amateur body builders. *International Journal of Sports Medicine*, **9**, 19-23.

Martikainen, H., Alen, M., Rahkila, P., & Vihko, R. (1986). Testicular responsiveness to human chorionic gonadotropin during transient hypogonadotropic hypogonadism induced by androgenic/anabolic steroids in power athletes. *Journal of Steroid Biochemistry*, **25**, 109-112.

McKillop, G., Ballantyne, F.C., Borland, W., & Ballantyne, D. (1989). Acute metabolic effects of exercise in bodybuilders using anabolic steroids. *British Journal of Sports Medicine*, **23**, 186-187.

O'Connor, J.S., Skinner, J.S., Baldini, F.D., & Einstein, M. (1990). Blood chemistry of current and previous anabolic steroid users. *Military Medicine*, **155**, 72-75.

Pope, H.G., Jr., & Katz, D.L. (1988). Affective and psychotic symptoms associated with anabolic steroid abuse. *American Journal of Psychiatry*, **145**, 487-490.

Rosse, R.B., & Deutsch, S.I. (1990). Hooked on hormones [Letter to the editor]. *Journal of the American Medical Association*, **263**, 2048-2049.

Scott, M.J. (1989). Cutaneous side effects of anabolic-androgenic steroid use. *Clinical Sports Medicine*, **1**, 5-16.

Tennant, F., Black, D.L., & Voy, R.O. (1988). Anabolic steroid dependence with opioid-type features [Letter to the editor]. *New England Journal of Medicine*, **319**, 578-579.

Wadler, G.I., & Hainline, B. (1989). *Drugs and the athlete*. Philadelphia: Davis.

Wilson, J.D., (1988). Androgen abuse by athletes. *Endocrine Reviews*, **9**, 181-199.

Urhausen, A., Holpes, R., & Kindermann, W. (1989). One- and two-dimensional echocardiography in bodybuilders using anabolic steroids. *European Journal of Applied Physiology*, **58**, 633-640.

Yesalis, C.E., Wright, J., & Lombardo, J.A. (1989). Anabolic-androgenic steroids: A synthesis of existing data and recommendations for future research. *Clinical Sports Medicine*, **1**, 109-134.

Zuliani, U., Bernardini, B., Catapano, A., Campana, M., Cerioli, G., & Spattini, M. (1988). Effects of anabolic steroids, testosterone, and HGH on blood lipids and echocardiographic parameters in body builders. *International Journal of Sports Medicine*, **10**, 62-66.

PART III

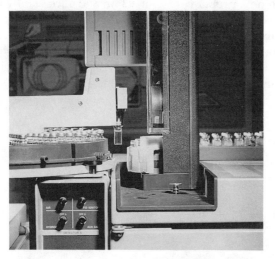

Testing and Societal Alternatives

The first 2 chapters that follow discuss drug testing in sport. Although testing involves a number of drugs besides anabolic steroids, significant attention is given to this topic because testing represents one of the primary strategies currently employed to combat drug use in sport. Politicians, fans, sport officials, the media, and even some athletes often appear to view drug testing as a "magic bullet" for this problem. Consequently, a critical analysis of the evolution, strengths, and frailties of drug testing is important.

Chapter 12 comes at the drug-testing issue from a political angle. It includes a candid discussion about the problems inherent in the current drug-testing system, such as secrecy, pharmacological warfare, loopholes, outlaw laboratories, false positives, and roadblocks to enforcement.

Chapter 13, on the other hand, looks at the scientific aspects of drug testing. Following a short history of drug testing, the chapter focuses on the metabolism of anabolic steroids, the technology involved in testing, the philosophy of testing, the costs of testing, and the circumventing of positive test results. The author also discusses the use of other substances to enhance performance, and future directions in drug testing.

251

To provide closure to this text but impetus for change, Charles Yesalis and James Wright consider societal alternatives to anabolic steroid use. In chapter 14, they point out that identifying potential solutions is easy, but that agreeing on a proper course of action and successfully completing it are difficult. They propose four alternatives for dealing with the use of anabolic steroids and other performance-enhancing drugs.

It is the contributors' hopes that the reader will have found this book to be not only a comprehensive resource on anabolic steroids but also a catalyst for individual and societal change.

CHAPTER 12

Evolution and Politics of Drug Testing

Jim Ferstle

Oh, what a tangled web we weave, when first we practice to deceive!

SIR WALTER SCOTT
Marmion, 1808

Drug testing of athletes is cloaked in mystery; it's a process that is conducted largely behind closed doors. This chapter contains a brief chronology of the origins of drug testing and the politics that affect the scientific process of examining body fluids for the presence of prohibited substances.

Origins

For nearly a century, sports administrators have tapped the expertise of laboratory scientists in an attempt to discover if athletes (or animal trainers) have attempted to enhance performance through the use of banned substances (Catlin, 1987). As the use of drugs has increased, so have their effects on the outcome of sporting events. Many athletes have become human guinea pigs, experimenting with all sorts of substances in an attempt to enhance their athletic prowess. Some of these experiments have resulted in death ("The death," 1988).

In 1960 a Danish cyclist died during the Olympics in Rome. His death was linked to the use of amphetamines. That same year, track athlete Dick Howard died, a death attributed to the use of "pep pills" (Wadler & Hainline, 1989). In the summer of 1967, British cyclist Tommy Simpson died during the Tour de France; amphetamines were found in his pockets and in his body. Governments and sports bodies reacted to the mounting pressure created by media reports of these incidents by passing legislation and instituting drug-testing programs (Donohoe & Johnson, 1986). By the end of 1967, the International Olympic Committee (IOC) had set up a medical commission, drafted rules prohibiting doping, and begun randomly testing athletes at both the 1968 winter and summer Games.

Drug use in the NFL was brought into the open in Dr. Arnold Mandell's (1976) book on the San Diego Chargers. Major league baseball players' use of pep pills was exposed by well-publicized Pittsburgh grand jury findings in 1985 (Donohoe & Johnson, 1986) and by Jim Bouton's (1970) book *Ball Four*. The NCAA was rocked by the drug-related death of a Clemson athlete and by the prosecution of several coaches who were distributing drugs to student athletes (Keisser, 1991).

Sports administrators' responses to these incidents were the same—the public announcement of an effort to rid the sport of drugs via testing and/ or drug-education programs. But the public image that was created of far-reaching programs that would control or wipe out drug use did not reflect reality.

Ollan Cassell, executive director of The Athletics Congress (TAC), voiced concern in 1991:

Of all the things in our sport that I have to deal with, the thing that scares me the most is drugs. . . . Our system is one of the best in the world. We want fair competition. . . . [But] we don't have a test for testosterone, for EPO [erythropoietin] or blood doping, or hGH. . . . [The testing system] is something we're still wrestling with. We still don't have all the answers. (Cassell, 1991)

History

The first "doping" tests were probably done using saliva. Concerned about drugged horses, the Austrian Jockey Club brought a Russian chemist to Vienna in 1910 to see if he could detect the presence of alkaloids in the saliva of race horses. Austrian professor Dr. Sigmund Frankel later developed a similar saliva test, and 218 such exams were conducted between 1910 and 1911 (IOC, 1973).

Although the testing of horses continued to develop and mature as a science, testing of human urine did not begin until the 1950s, when the Italian soccer and cycling federations requested that the FMSI (Italian Medical Sports Federation) laboratory in Florence test soccer players and cyclists. After the 1960 Summer Olympics in Rome, CONI (the Italian National Olympic Committee) joined forces with FMSI to set up a second drug-testing lab in Rome (Gasbarrone & Rosati, 1988).

At various times during the 1950s, sports medicine groups met in Austria and Germany to hold symposiums or inquiries into the problem, and in 1959, the International Sports Medicine Congresses focused on the issue at their meeting in Paris. Dr. Manfred Donike (Donike et al., 1988), director of the Institute for Biochemistry laboratory in Cologne, speaking at an International Athletic Foundation (IAF)–sponsored conference on doping in sport in 1987, traced the beginnings of "modern" drug testing. "Starting about 1960, the modern techniques of analytical chemistry, especially chromotography, provided the possibility to detect more and more dope agents or their metabolites in biological fluids, preferentially in urine," said Donike (Donike et al., 1988, p. 53).

In 1959, the Association Nationale d'Education Physique formed a doping commission in France. In 1962, FMSI organized a doping inquiry, and the IOC passed a resolution condemning doping. On September 30, 1962, the Austrian government, through the federal ministry of education, set up a doping commission. These organizations passed their own regulations that included sanctions against those found guilty of doping offenses (IOC, 1973).

In January 1963, at a meeting in Strasbourg, France, the Council of Europe defined doping as follows:

The administering or use of substances in any form alien to the body or of physiological substances in abnormal amounts and with abnormal methods by healthy persons with the exclusive aim of attaining an artificial and unfair increase of performance in competition. Furthermore, various psychological measures to increase performance in sports must be regarded as doping. (IOC, 1973)

All the organizations involved in the issue struggled with the dual problem of defining doping and establishing what constituted proof of a doping offense. Considerable time was spent drafting language that was acceptable to everyone. For example, one concern was the difficulty of discriminating between doping and legitimate medical treatment with a substance that could improve performance; so in November 1963 in Madrid, the European Doping Colloquium passed an amendment to the original doping definition to address this problem:

Where treatment with medicine must be undergone, which as a result of its nature or dosage is capable of raising physical capability above the normal level, such treatment must be considered as doping and shall rule out eligibility for competition. (IOC, 1973)

The group included with this amendment the first "official" list of banned substances. It included narcotics; amine stimulants; alkaloids, such as strychnine and ephedrine; and all analeptic agents, respiratory tonics, and certain hormones (IOC, 1973).

By November 1964, the first known government-sponsored, antidoping legislation was proposed by members of the French Senate. The law forbade the misuse of pharmacological substances for doping, and it levied fines, disqualifications, and jail sentences of up to 1 year for the offenders. The law was passed, went into effect in 1965, and was followed that same year by a similar antidoping act passed in Belgium (IOC, 1973).

All these proposals, position statements, definitions, and pieces of legislation were difficult to implement, however, because of various legal entanglements. The measures conflicted with other laws or international agreements or were difficult to enforce because of the lack of clear guidelines or regulations.

Even something seemingly simple, such as agreement regarding what substances should be on the banned list, was difficult to achieve. Into this breach stepped the IOC, which established its medical commission in 1967 under the leadership of Prince Alexandre de Merode of Belgium, a former cyclist who after becoming aware of the doping problem in his sport began to work within the sports organizations to set up a doping control program in the 1950s.

The International Amateur Athletic Federation (IAAF) also formed a subcommittee on doping under its medical commission and pioneered the process of accrediting drug-testing labs. In 1978, the IAAF medical commission subcommission drafted a paper titled "Standardization of Analytical Procedures and Quality Tests for Doping Control Laboratories" (Donike et al., 1988).

These rules were adopted at the IAAF medical commission's annual meeting in March 1979 in Berlin and at the IAAF Council in April 1979 in Dakar, Senegal. In 1980, the medical commission of the IOC drafted their own requirements for accreditation. Laboratories passing this test are required to be reaccredited every 2 years. This method of certifying laboratories was begun in 1985 (Donike, 1988). Through increased testing and further development of the laboratory accreditation process, Prince de Merode and his colleagues on the IOC medical commission developed what has become the industry standard in doping control (Dubin, 1990).

The IOC medical commission has encouraged the sports governing bodies, under the umbrella of the IOC, to standardize the list of banned substances. It has supported economically and educationally the development of drug-testing laboratories at various Olympic venues, such as Montreal, Calgary, and Los Angeles (Hatton & Catlin, 1987).

Researchers from the Chelsea Laboratory in London developed methods of testing for anabolic steroids in the early 1970s, and unofficial testing for the substances was conducted at the Summer Olympics in Munich in 1972. The first official tests for the presence of anabolic steroids were done in Montreal in 1976 (Hatton & Catlin, 1987).

Dr. Donike, whose laboratory performed the testing at the 1972 Munich Games, noted that finding banned substances was only part of the job. Sport governing bodies were also concerned about how quickly drug test results could be obtained.

The ability to detect dope agents covers only one part of the problem. Analysis capacity and turnover rate between

> receipt of the samples and reporting the results are the other important factors, especially at major events. The first occasion where dope analysis of a larger number of urine samples was realized were the Olympic Games 1972, Munich, when 2,079 samples were analyzed within 14 days. After this demonstration, dope control with all its implications was accepted by the International Sports Federations and Authorities and introduced at major championships and other important events (Donike et al., 1988, p. 53).

Prior to the Games in Montreal in 1976, Dr. Donike and his colleagues at the Federal Institute for Sports Science published an information brochure titled *The Doping Controls in Montreal*. Its intent was to "thoroughly inform both the athletes and their physicians, coaches, and counsellors about the medical regulations of the IOC" (Kirsch, 1988, p. 220). A chapter titled "How to protect against unjustified doping charges" was included. About 7,500 copies of this brochure were printed and distributed.

This booklet was reprinted in 1980 and 1984, and about 25,000 copies were distributed during that time. A companion piece, *Doping, Information Brochure for Athletes and Coaches*, was published in 1986. This publication, with the financial assistance of the IAAF, was also reprinted in English; the others were only available in German (Kirsch, 1988). A similar publication was distributed in the United States at about the same time by TAC and in England by the British Amateur Athletic Board (BAAB).

The British began testing at international competitions held in Great Britain in 1975. Under the leadership of Sir Arthur Gold, Dr. Raymond Brooks of St. Thomas Hospital, and Dr. David Cowan and Dr. Arnold Beckett at the Chelsea Lab, research was undertaken into many of the problem areas of sport drug testing: detection of anabolic steroids, hGH, HCG, and blood doping (Bottomley, 1988).

In 1985, the Sports Council of England provided financial assistance for a pilot program of out-of-season testing of British athletes eligible for international selection. The BAAB began a program of random, out-of-competition testing in 1986 (Bottomley, 1988). Norway and Sweden also developed out-of-competition testing programs and began to coordinate efforts between the athletic governing bodies and their federal governments in an attempt to control the importation of banned substances (Norman, 1988). Customs officials in Norway confiscated 200,000 tablets in 1986, 5,000 of which were identified as narcotics and 20,000 as anabolic steroids (Norman, 1988).

De Merode and others on the IOC medical commission struggled to establish uniformity in a system rife with national and international differences. At the World Conference on Anti-Doping in Sport in June 1988, de Merode said,

It is totally unacceptable that in one country you can take this drug and in another country you cannot. . . . (Boswell, 1988) We need common legislation. The premises of doping control have been laid. . . . There is a lack of harmonization between sports federations and politicians. (Stuart, 1988)

Laws against doping wouldn't work for everyone, however, as illustrated by the comments of another delegate to that conference, Dr. Eduardo de Rose of Brazil. "We will not use legislation because we are not used to following legislation," said de Rose when asked if Norway's approach would work in his country. "We have a law against everything and we do everything" (Hynes, 1988, June 29).

Later in 1988, officials of the United States Olympic Committee (USOC) and the then–Soviet Union began work to establish a cooperative drug testing program between the two countries. A pact was signed in 1989 and others were invited to join in the coalition, but the response was lukewarm at best. Canada, Italy, Czechoslovakia, and what was then West Germany joined the superpowers in a meeting in Moscow in October 1989, but East Germany and other nations did not. Representatives from U.S. and Soviet laboratories visited one another's labs and exchanged information in an attempt to achieve a standard of operation in their testing systems ("Doping tests," 1989; Warshaw, 1989).

Due to the different economic and political conditions in various countries, IOC lab directors acknowledge that the capabilities of various labs within the IOC system vary. Well-funded labs in Cologne or Los Angeles, for example, have more resources than a lab in Czechoslovakia or Moscow (Catlin, 1991). Thus, it has been suggested that a two-track accreditation system be implemented within the IOC, with which one standard is applied to the established laboratories and another standard to those who do not have the resources.

In 1990, TAC proposed to the IAAF that a system of challenge testing be implemented, for which each nation would choose a number of athletes from another country who would be subject to an unannounced test (Chriss, 1990). Neither the U.S.-Soviet program, nor the challenge testing concept, has been implemented.

The NFL had begun testing its players for drugs in training camps in 1982 (Demak & Kirshenbaum, 1990) but didn't test for anabolic steroids until 1987 (Forbes, 1989). By 1990 that program had expanded to include some random testing every 6 weeks.

In 1986 the NCAA began to develop a drug-testing program. This program is tightly controlled by the NCAA, and at first it only included limited testing at or before major bowl games or championships. It has since expanded to include some random testing of athletes and is bolstered by separate testing programs conducted by the universities (C.E. Yesalis, personal communication, 1991).

The Men's International Professional Tennis Council agreed in November 1985 that tennis players would submit to urinalysis at two of the five major tournaments. This initial testing was only for "social drugs," such as amphetamines and cocaine ("Drug tests sought," 1987). The program was later expanded in some situations to include anabolic steroids, and the players who competed in the 1988 Olympics were subject to IOC testing (Wadler & Hainline, 1989).

TAC, the governing body for track and field in the United States, established an out-of-competition, random drug testing program in 1989. A year later, TAC also banned "for life" a prominent Southern California track coach, Chuck DeBus, amid allegations that he regularly urged athletes he trained to use performance-enhancing substances (National Athletics Board of Review of The Athletics Congress, 1990).

The NFL was apparently forced to remove its director of drug testing, Dr. Forest Tennant, in 1990 after a Washington, DC, television reporter and an article in *Sports Illustrated* suggested that the NFL drug-testing program was not being properly administered (Glauber, 1990). Tennant was also embroiled in a controversy surrounding the "positive" drug test of stock car driver Tim Richmond. Tennant maintained that accusations that he was enlisted by the National Association of Stock Car Racers (NASCAR) to produce a positive test from Richmond were false ("Richmond-Tennant," 1990).

Dr. Bo Berglund and the researchers at the Karolinska Institute in Sweden led the way in the development of a test for blood doping, but even they admit that it can only detect the practice if a person is using someone else's blood. The first blood tests specifically designed to detect blood doping were performed at the world cross-country skiing championships in 1988 (Videman, 1989).

In 1991, the IOC medical commission recommended that blood tests be used at the Olympics, possibly starting with the Winter Games in 1994. Although IOC officials insisted that such a program could be implemented, others questioned whether the considerable legal, AIDS-related, and cultural issues involved with such a program could be circumvented to allow full implementation of blood testing for drugs as well as blood doping (Wilson, 1991).

Secrecy and Credibility

Thanks to the efforts of a legion of dedicated scientists, physicians, athletes, coaches, and sports administrators, sports drug testing has advanced from "ground zero" to a fairly sophisticated industry. However, two aspects of the system still appear to hinder its development and the public perception of its effectiveness. The cloak of secrecy that surrounds all testing and the fact that sports-governing bodies still control nearly every aspect of the testing process have caused some to question the credibility of the system's enforcement process.

The Dubin Inquiry report blasted the IOC's accreditation process because of the fact that the people who do the accrediting are also directors of some of the laboratories being accredited. Numerous athletes, coaches, and officials have charged that drug-testing rules are some times selectively enforced. Others contend that the system is easy to circumvent, either because there is no random testing or because the sample collection process is easy to subvert. In a 1991 speech, Robert Armstrong, Chief Council to Canadian Justice Minister Charles Dubin (who directed the Dubin Inquiry), addressed these concerns:

While the concept of a universal standard for laboratory accreditation is to be applauded, the present system of accreditation is, in my view, subject to a serious problem of conflict of interest. The problem arises because some of the members of the IOC subcommission who determine which laboratories will be accredited and which laboratories will have their accreditation revoked also operate their own laboratories, which are accredited by the IOC. They have the ability to create a monopoly and an unfair price system. . . .

To use a phrase from English common law, it is important not only that justice be done, but that justice appear to be done. Unless an athlete has full right of appeal, including the right and ability to challenge the scientific validity of the drug test, he or she will be denied a full right of review of any positive test. Chief Justice Dubin therefore recommended "that the grounds of appeal against a positive doping control test result be expanded to include challenges to the scientific validity of the test." (Armstrong, 1991, pp. 24-25)

Dr. Donald Catlin, director of the IOC-accredited laboratory at the University of California-Los Angeles (UCLA), disputed the Canadians' conclusions (Catlin, 1991). He said that the Dubin Inquiry only considered limited testimony, mainly confined to the Canadian system, and that it is unfair to brand the entire IOC system as deficient based on this examination. He said he believes that the IOC system does allow for adequate review of tests. It is not a perfect system, he acknowledged, but it is the best that has yet been developed.

To merely look at alleged shortcomings ignores the development of a sophisticated analytical system that must operate in a worldwide arena that is not immune from politics. Dr. Catlin compared the difficulty of drug-testing negotiations to the nuclear arms race. Trying to develop a uniform drug-testing system that is immune from politics or free from imperfections is like attempting to rid the world of thermonuclear devices, he said.

Dr. Robert Voy, former director of sports medicine for the USOC, was skeptical. He didn't criticize the scientists who operate the labs but rather the sports administrators who are charged with imposing sanctions based on the test results. He addressed this in his book, *Drugs, Sport, and Politics*:

Allowing national governing bodies, international federations, and national Olympic Committees such as the United States Olympic Committee to govern the testing process to ensure fair play in sport is terribly ineffective. In a sense, it is like having the fox guard the henhouse.

There is simply too much money involved in international sports today. One needs to understand that the officials in charge of operating sport at the amateur level need world-class performances to keep their businesses rolling forward. . . . The athletes and officials realize this, so they're willing to do whatever it takes to win. And sometimes that means turning their backs on the drug problem. (Voy & Deeter, 1991, p. 101)

Dr. Voy is not alone in making this charge. Irish cyclist-turned-journalist Paul Kimmage, in writing *A Rough Ride: An Insight Into ProCycling*, was equally blunt in his criticism of the cycling sports authorities and their attitudes regarding enforcement of drug-testing rules.

The men in power want a solution all right, but a painless one. . . . The grapevine is a dreadfully frustrating source of knowledge. Facts are often distorted, but there is no

> smoke without fire. I've heard stories of corruption that would make you ill. Of race organizers giving the green light to champions to take anything they want. Of urine samples that never reach laboratories. The temptation by those on the make is to cover up and not own up. But by not owning up we will continue to suck in the innocents and spit out the victims. (Kimmage, 1990, pp. 185-186)

Former French Open champion Yannick Noah openly questioned the tennis testing program's effectiveness. He said that testing was only done for public relations, not to catch cheaters. "I don't think they are going to find anything," he said. "They don't really want to. If they wanted to discover something they would test every week" ("Wimbledon-drugs," 1990).

It is not merely rumor that taints the system. In sworn testimony given during the doping case of U.S. discus thrower Ben Plucknett in 1981, Dr. Beckett acknowledged that some of the urine samples at the 1976 Winter Olympics had been tampered with. Testing had to be halted at those Games because of the incident, Beckett said (Plucknett v. TAC/USA, 1982).

The official report of the IOC issued after the 1984 Olympics in Los Angeles and a scientific paper published by Dr. Catlin and his associates at the UCLA lab that did the testing also yielded some discrepancies (Catlin, Kammerer, Hatton, et al., 1987; Dubin, 1990; Los Angeles Olympic Organizing Committee, 1985; Wadler & Hainline, 1989). When asked about the fact that the number of positives announced and the number reported in Dr. Catlin's paper did not match, Prince de Merode told a newspaper reporter in February 1988 that the IOC had waited until a medical commission meeting in November 1988 in Mexico to make public the other positive results (de Merode, 1988).

Dr. Voy, for one, still wonders what happened. "The numbers don't add up," he said (Voy, unpublished interview, 1988).

Part of the problem rests with the fact that an "analytically positive test" may not serve as grounds for sanctions. At the Olympics, as at other major championships, a medical panel is enlisted to review the laboratory results. This process can create the appearance of a cover-up.

In Helsinki in 1983 at the IAAF world track-and-field championships, Dr. Donike admitted in testimony before the Dubin Inquiry that some of the A-samples appeared to have excess levels of testosterone. Upon review, however, the medical panel decided not to test the B-samples. When an athlete provides a urine sample for testing, the sample is poured from the bottle in which it was collected into an A-sample bottle and a B-sample bottle. The A-sample is opened and tested at the laboratory. The B-sample is not tested unless a banned substance is found in the A-sample. The athlete has the right to be present when the B-sample is opened and tested. This system was created to help protect against tampering or sabotage of an athlete's specimen (Buffrey & Parrish, 1989).

If there is evidence of tampering, or if the seals on the bottles have been accidentally broken prior to testing, most organizations' drug-testing rules mandate that the test results are invalid and cannot be used to sanction an athlete. Because this process is not open to independent scrutiny, the perception has been created that some samples can be treated differently than others (Buffery & Parrish, 1989).

For example, in 1988 10 athletes were banned from the Summer Olympics in Seoul for flunking drug tests. Dr. Jongsei Park, the director of the drug-testing lab in Seoul, told a reporter for the *New York Times* that "as many as 20 other athletes tested positive and were not disqualified" (Janofsky & Alfano, 1988). Dr. Arne Ljungqvist, head of the IAAF medical commission and a member of the IOC medical commission, disputed the use of the term *positive* in the Seoul cases.

Dr. Park also denied that there was any cover-up of positive tests when he was asked about the story at an IAF conference in Monte Carlo in 1989. He noted that four of the positive tests were cases in which HCG was detected in the urine samples, and four others were positive tests for marijuana, a substance not banned by the IOC. At least two of the urines containing HCG were from pregnant women, said Dr. Park (Park, 1989).

The IOC provided a summary of the drug testing at Seoul that listed four categories:

- the 10 positive tests,
- 6 "cases discussed and determined as not positive,"
- 3 IOC "control" samples—samples with known quantities of banned substances sent to the lab to test the lab's ability to make the proper analysis, and
- 15 samples that were studied "upon the request of the IOC Medical Commission" for "additional scientific research" (IOC, 1989).

An Associated Press news story quoted Dr. Ljungqvist:

It is completely wrong to refer to those cases as positive. The results of an analysis is not like a sheet of paper which says positive, but an analytical data which requires a specialist evaluation. In most cases, it's quite clear that a sample contains a banned substance and in other cases it's not.

But there are cases which are difficult to decide upon and require careful study. Some of those cases may then be judged as not positive and will therefore not be reported. This is, in all probability, what happened in some cases in Seoul like it happened in any other major competition. ("IOC-drugs," 1988)

At the IAF-sponsored conference on drugs in sport in Monte Carlo in 1989, Dr. Ljungqvist and Dr. Beckett were grilled by the media on this perceptual problem. They steadfastly denied that there had ever been a cover-up of positive drug test results. When asked if the drug test records—test results with ID numbers attached, no identifying names— would ever be made public to squash the speculation and put an end to the rumors, both replied that they didn't believe that was possible (Beckett & Ljungqvist, 1989).

This inability of the system to be open to independent scrutiny provides the most ammunition to its critics. As long as there is secrecy, doubt about what really happened can be propagated. Until the veil is lifted, the system will remain an easy target for those who want to use this issue as a club.

Politics and Pharmacological Warfare

Armstrong further criticized the IOC at the International Symposium on Sport and Law in Monte Carlo in 1991:

The IOC and its Medical Commission have known for years that testing for anabolic steroids at the time of competition was a virtual waste of time in terms of providing effective deterrent for their use during training periods. . . . There had been a failure of leadership among our sporting governing organizations, both at the national and international level. If you examine the Dubin Report carefully, I think you will agree that our sport leaders have let us down. If you are going to lead, you must lead from the head of the line. You must be out front. You cannot lead by reacting after the fact. (Armstrong, 1991, pp. 19-20)

De Merode and Hans Skaset, the president of Norway's Confederation of Sport, pointed out at the World Conference on Anti-Doping in Sport in 1988 that leadership in an international arena is not easy to achieve. Implementing an international plan is not as simple as believing you have the appropriate solution; it also involves negotiating with leaders of sometimes hostile nations to accomplish an often not-so-common goal; as Skaset pointed out:

You have all sorts of mistrust mixed in with this; you have the East-West dimension. . . . If we could have something like an INF treaty between the Soviet Union, the German Democratic Republic and the United States, then they would have to patrol each other. . . .

Too much money is used on testing that everybody knows about. It has very little effect—or no effect. . . . You can produce statistics showing that we have tested 35,000 persons in one year, as the International Olympic Committee did in 1987, and only some eight or 10 were caught. But that is, of course, because everybody knows the game. You have to have a system that is not protective of your athletes. If it is you're cheating. You are corrupting yourself. (Hynes, 1988)

De Merode added,

It's absolutely necessary to do it, to have random tests during competition, but through training as well. It's the next step we have to pass, but it's only possible if the concept is acceptable to everybody. . . . You cannot tell an international federation you cannot do this. We can only tell them of the problem. ("Down on dope," 1988, p. 80)

De Merode acknowledged that the IOC medical commission is not the most powerful lobbying force within the IOC. As history indicates, reform in the drug-testing system usually follows a crisis.

The drug testers don't operate in a vacuum. In addition to dealing with the politicians and legislators, they have to fight a pharmacological war with athletes and their advisers, who are constantly attempting to stay one step ahead of the laboratories. Charlie Francis was Ben Johnson's coach from 1981 until 1988. He was nicknamed by some of his peers as "Charlie the chemist," not because he had a degree in biochemistry but because Francis knew not only how to coach but also about drugs and the drug-testing system (Denton, 1989).

When he was coaching and after Johnson was caught, Francis was kept up-to-date on the latest in sports pharmacology by a wide array of individuals operating in and behind the scenes in track and field. From undetectable anabolic steroids to masking agents, Francis heard stories about all forms of substances athletes were taking in an attempt to beat the drug-testing system. New substances included clenbuterol, a supposed steroid substitute; syndocarb, a stimulant that was at one time unavailable to laboratory testers and, therefore, undetectable; and a substance called lipoplex that is supposed to metabolize the metabolites of a steroid so that its by-products will not be recognized on a drug screen as those of a banned substance (Francis, 1991). Athletes were also taking gonadotropin-releasing hormones in an attempt to balance their endocrine profiles; as a result, their profiles looked normal and the athletes could not be sanctioned by any new test that used these profiles.

Dr. Mauro Di Pasquale (1991) discussed this in the newsletter *Drugs in Sports*:

In the past few years there has been such an emphasis on the use of anabolic steroids that few people, other than the athletes themselves, have noticed the quiet revolution that has been occurring. While athletes are still using anabolic steroids (there has been little decrease in the use of anabolic steroids by the more pharmacologically sophisticated athletes), most are making extensive use of other compounds for the purposes of enhancing their performance, with or without the concomitant use of anabolic steroids.

These compounds are used as ergogenic aids, masking agents to conceal the use of anabolic steroids, and therapeutic agents to deal with the side effects of anabolic steroid use. Many of these compounds are either not detectable or are not tested for, further increasing the incentive for their use. As well many athletes are looking for alternative compounds because of the scarcity of and the uncertainty over the authenticity and quality of present black market anabolic steroids. (p. 2)

Each of these forms of subterfuge may fail if the lab knows what to look for, which is one reason why IOC lab directors are so concerned about secrecy and why those attempting to beat the system are constantly scouring the medical journals to uncover those secrets. A product called Defend, manufactured by southern California bodybuilder Vince Bovino, has been advertised as a masking agent, a substance that will foil a drug test by masking the presence of a banned substance in the urine (Biggane, 1991).

Analysis of the product has revealed that it is merely glucose, which has no known masking properties (Kammerer, 1991). Bovino is touting its benefit to the press, but others contend he's just out to make a buck.

Does masking work or is this merely the case of an enterprising individual attempting to take advantage of a new niche in the marketplace? In the mid-1980s athletes used probenecid to block the excretion of banned substances (Catlin & Hatton, 1991). They diluted their urine, used catheters, and hid bags of "clean" urine on or in their bodies in an attempt to beat the system. German sprint champions Katrin Krabbe and Silke Gladisch Moller and quarter-miler Grit Breuer were suspended in February of 1992 by their federation for allegedly attempting to subvert the testing system by hiding clean urine in condom-like rubber pouches inserted in their vaginas ("Von vorn bis hinten belogen," 1992). These athletes were sanctioned after laboratory analysis of their urine revealed that all three samples had been provided by the same person, prompting the German magazine *Der Spiegel* to comment that the three had attempted to subvert the process by using a "urine cocktail."

The German track and field federation also revealed it suspected that Krabbe and Breuer had used a similar technique in July 1991 because two samples provided by the athletes at that time were also from one individual, according to the results of the laboratory analysis. It has been rumored that these and other techniques are used extensively by athletes to beat the testing system. Nobody really knows how often they succeed.

In the 1990s, athletes are resorting to polypharmacy—use of a wide variety of substances—to beat the system (DiPasquale, 1991). The mystery remains: How much of this pharmacological competition is fact and how much is fiction?

Loopholes

IOC-accredited labs have had an unblemished record in the analysis of drug samples. They have waded through the morass of identifying a veritable laundry list of drugs that can be taken by athletes and have dealt with the problems of masking agents, diuretics, and compounds that closely resemble banned substances, such as birth control pills. Only three cases, the 1987 suspension of Swiss distance runner Sandra Gasser, the 1988 positive test of U.S. swimmer Angel Meyers (Martino), and the 1990 case of 400-m world-record holder Harry "Butch" Reynolds, have gone to court to challenge the science of the drug tests.

Testimony by Dr. David Black (1991) in the Reynolds case created enough doubt about the validity of the test in the minds of a U.S. federal arbitrator and a three-member TAC panel that they ruled in favor of Reynolds. Dr. Black's review of the test done in an IOC-accredited lab in Paris raised several questions about the accuracy and interpretation of Reynolds's test data. Doubts were also raised about the "chain of custody" when a lawyer for Reynolds demonstrated that the seal on the "envopak" that contains the urine sample could be "picked" with a dental pick.

This flaw in the chain of custody did not prove that Reynolds's sample had been tampered with, but it created doubt about the system that is supposed to ensure against tampering. Each sample is collected in a beaker that is selected by the athlete. After the athlete has been observed urinating into the beaker, the urine is poured into two bottles (these are the A- and B-samples). The bottles are marked with a code number, sealed, and sent to the laboratory in an envopak that is also sealed with a tab that has a coded number on it. Any serious breach of this chain-of-custody process can be grounds for invalidating the analytical results of the tests on the bottles' contents.

The conclusion we reach in this case is based upon evidence presented in two primary areas: (1) chain of custody and (2) laboratory procedure and data analysis. None of these issues in and of themselves would have been sufficient to allow us to reach the conclusion that Mr. Reynolds was not guilty of the charge against him. Taken together, however, there is a strong case that can be made which leaves too much doubt to find against him. (TAC Doping Control Review Board, 1991, p. 7)

Thus, although scientific issues were involved in the disposition of the Reynolds case, the main issues on which the case turned were procedural (i.e., problems in the chain of custody). Such is also the case in the other area in which athletes have successfully overturned analytically positive tests: through the appeals process of a sport's governing body. Doriane Lambelet, an attorney and a nationally ranked 800-m runner who was instrumental in drafting comprehensive legislation for TAC's out-of-competition testing program and revamping TAC's current rules in 1989, provided a revealing commentary on the rules that governed the drug-testing appeals process in track and field.

"It appeared that whoever drafted these rules was either not very bright or that they wanted people to get off," said Lambelet (1989) about the old rules. "The way the legislation was drafted, there were plenty of loopholes." Several cases in the United States that illustrated some of the loopholes Lambelet was talking about prompted her and others to seek changes in the drug-testing appeals process after athletes successfully challenged lab results.

In 1987, U.S. discus thrower John Powell was informed that a sample he allegedly provided after the TAC championships had tested positive for nandrolone. Powell appealed, stating that TAC could not prove that the sample was his because of irregularities in the sample collection and labeling (Almond, 1990).

A key piece of evidence in Powell's appeal was the fact that the documents accompanying his sample rendered the test invalid, according to the members of the appeals panel. Others pointed out that the mislabeling could have easily been intentional and should not have invalidated the test (USOC, 1987). As a result of this case, TAC rules were changed so that a labeling error would not automatically invalidate a positive result (Lambelet, 1989). Other TAC cases also resulted in a new TAC rule regarding testosterone.

Successful Appeals

In 1989, shot-putter August Wolf and pole vaulter Billy Olsen were informed that samples they provided at the TAC indoor championships had higher than the allowed limit for testosterone. Both appealed and presented witnesses challenging the validity of the testosterone test. Their appeals were successful and neither was disciplined (TAC, 1989).

Subsequently a rule was passed at the 1989 TAC convention stating that a testosterone-to-epitestosterone (T/E) ratio of over 6:1 would be considered a positive result and the onus was on the athlete to prove that his or her ratio was not the result of drug use (TAC, 1990). This doctrine of guilty until proven innocent has held up, even though challenged by Butch Reynolds and shot put world-record holder Randy Barnes.

Both contended that TAC's rules violated the U.S. constitution, which ensures that a person is considered innocent until proven guilty. The burden is usually on the prosecutor to prove that the accused is guilty, rather than the accused having to demonstrate that the charges are false (TAC Doping Control Review Board, 1991). Reynolds won his appeal in the United States; Barnes did not.

The U.S. judicial philosophy of innocent until proven guilty contributed to Reynolds's winning his TAC appeal but may not be upheld in

Europe, where the philosophy is "guilty until proven innocent," as the Gasser case illustrated. Gasser was also found innocent by her federation, but she lost her case in the British courts, which ruled that she failed to prove her innocence (Gasser v. Stinson, 1988).

This legal confusion amply illustrates some of the difficulties encountered by sports administrators and athletes who are forced to litigate what appears to be an analytically positive drug test.

Problems With Testosterone

The TAC testosterone cases were not the only cases in which athletes have created doubt in the minds of appeals panels regarding an analytically positive drug test. Basketball player Stacey Augmon and hockey player Corey Millen were able to convince the USOC that their elevated testosterone levels were not the result of doping.

Millen played for the U.S. Olympic hockey team in 1984 and 1988, and Augmon played basketball for the 1988 U.S. team. Millen was banned by the International Ice Hockey Federation in 1989 because of his over-the-limit testosterone ("Millen barred," 1989), but Augmon successfully appealed his over-the-limit testosterone test results before an IOC medical panel at the 1988 Summer Olympics in Seoul (Almond, 1990). Both argued that their bodies produced naturally high levels of testosterone that caused their ratios to be outside the 6-to-1 IOC limit. The ice hockey federation, however, refused to accept Millen's defense.

The dispositions of these cases illustrate the difficulty that scientists and governing bodies have with substances that are naturally produced. Testosterone, hGH, and erythropoietin are banned substances that the human body produces naturally. Comprehensive studies of what constitutes normal levels of these substances have not yet been conducted (Catlin & Hatton, 1991).

The studies by IOC labs have been primarily on athletes; only in recent years have these labs started to test other populations to validate or alter the 6:1 ratio that they currently use as the guideline for determining an analytically positive test for doping using testosterone. The NCAA considered raising the ratio above 6:1 in 1990 and the IOC considered lowering the ratio to 4:1 (Ferstle, 1991). These examples illustrate the intensity of the scientific debate on the subject.

This situation has allowed athletes to create doubt about the validity of the test for testosterone and opened a rather large loophole in the testing system. Dr. Donike has advocated backing up positive results through the use of endocrine profiles, such as the one used in the Johnson case in Seoul to refute Johnson's contention that his drinks were spiked ("Update," 1989).

The endocrine profile has been controversial within the drug-testing community for the same reason the other natural substances cause problems—there is a lack of controlled scientific studies to determine normal and abnormal levels of the substances being identified and measured. But the international weight-lifting federation has embraced the concept and has publicly announced that it will use the test process to weed out drug users in the sport.

Advised of the use of profiles, however, athletes have begun using substances such as gonadotropin-releasing hormones to give themselves "normal" profiles.

Outlaw Laboratories

Another problem the sports drug-testing laboratories face is competition, not for contracts to test events but from tests done by commercial labs that protect athletes from being caught. The IOC lab directors call them "outlaw laboratories." These labs will test the urine of anyone who pays the fee (Catlin & Moses, 1989).

The testing is done anonymously and no sanctions are imposed. Athletes use the services, for example, to determine their T/E ratios so they can stay just under the detection limit of the IOC tests. A more serious example of this behavior has been the revelation in the Soviet and German press of the pretesting of Olympic athletes by laboratories in those countries to make sure athletes attending international competitions were clean (Harvey, 1990; Starcevic, 1990).

In 1984 the USOC allowed U.S. athletes to anonymously send urine samples to the UCLA lab for testing. USOC officials said that the program was designed to allow the UCLA lab to gain experience handling and analyzing drug samples but later admitted that the program was a mistake and that athletes used the program to learn about their clearance times (Patrick, 1989; Puffer, 1988). Craig Kammerer, who was the assistant director of the laboratory in 1984, said that lab staff were not given the same explanation as the public by the USOC:

> We never heard that. We were told that positive results from the tests at the Olympic trials would be grounds for keeping people off the team. And some people did lose their place on the Olympic team in 1984, but we saw more than the number who weren't allowed to compete. (Kammerer, 1991)

In response to the actions of the "rogue labs," de Merode announced in May 1988 the promulgation of a code of ethics for IOC-accredited labs. The code forbids IOC labs from doing testing for individuals ("Labs under," 1988). This has not stopped athletes from seeking such assistance. IOC lab directors are called regularly by individuals seeking testing. Some non-IOC labs openly offer the service. Augie Wolf was actively soliciting business for one such lab in 1990, sending a prospectus offering anonymous testing at a lab in northern California (Moses, 1989).

Some IOC lab directors snicker at this process, noting that representatives from these rogue labs have accompanied athletes who have produced positive A-samples to observe the testing of the B-samples. The "outlaw lab" operators are attempting to discover what process the IOC lab uses that allows the athlete to test negative on the outlaw-lab test but positive in the IOC-accredited lab (Catlin, 1991).

Beating the System

Still, athletes will try almost anything to beat the system. They will consult with so-called "steroid gurus" for ways to beat the tests or for access to the latest undetectable substances. They will have a teammate or friend urinate for them and switch samples. They will be tipped off as to when the tests will be conducted so they will be "clean" (Bedell, 1991).

They will inject epitestosterone to foil the tests that measure the testosterone-to-epitestosterone ratio. Or they will use vinegar, salt, bleach, WD-40 lubricant, hydrogen peroxide, or ammonia in an attempt to produce a negative sample (Bedell, 1991). Catheters and condoms have also been used to substitute or store urine that is emptied into the collection bottle at the appropriate time.

And, if all this fails, athletes will use more extreme measures. One American athlete "accidentally" dropped his B-sample bottle in an attempt to void his positive test. When the bottle didn't break, he picked it up and threw it, smashing the bottle and voiding the test. He could not be suspended for a failed drug test but could be sanctioned for a deliberate attempt to subvert the system (Ferstle, 1991).

False Positives

Lab work that is not up to IOC standards can also produce false positives, as was illustrated by three recent cases. In 1989, Norwegian javelin thrower Trine (Solberg) Hattestad was convicted by her federation and the IAAF of flunking a drug test at the European Cup meet in Brussels. The IAAF later reversed the conviction and decertified the lab that did the test.

Hattestad sued the Norwegian federation and was awarded a $50,000 judgment ("Solberg wins," 1990).

In early 1991, the female member of a Soviet pairs team was also accused of producing a positive test. The result was leaked after an A-sample tested in an uncertified lab in Sofia, Bulgaria, was deemed to be positive for excessive testosterone. The B-sample analysis done in Cologne was negative. The skating federation was reprimanded and told not to use noncertified labs for its testing (Zanca, 1991).

The conviction of a Yugoslavian long jumper at the 1990 European championships was also recently overturned by the IAAF ("Bilac back," 1991). These cases illustrate that quality control is a major issue in drug testing. The competence of a laboratory can often determine whether an athlete is judged guilty or innocent.

Funding

In effect, the sports governing bodies fund this cottage industry of sports dope testing. The money does not come in the form of grants for scientific research on drugs in sport, but rather as fees for analyzing samples. In effect, therefore, the drug-testing system is monetarily driven by testing.

Many sports administrators believe that merely the threat of testing would deter athletes from using drugs. These administrators ignored the advice of many of the emerging pioneers in the field of sports drug testing, such as Brooks and Beckett of London, Donike of the Cologne Laboratory, and Dr. Robert Dugal from Montreal, by adopting a minimalist approach to drug testing. They only funded tests during competitions and announced the testing in advance (Dubin, 1990).

Almost from the beginning, therefore, a gap existed between what many scientists advised and what sports authorities were willing to fund or enforce.

Legal and Enforcement Roadblocks

Whenever stiff penalties were proposed, they were often opposed by those citing legal objections. For example, several individuals challenged the NCAA's drug-testing programs on the grounds that they violated individuals' rights in the United States (Almond, 1989; "Court backs," 1988; "Update," 1989; Wong, 1988).

Many of the same arguments were made when individuals proposed out-of-competition, random testing of athletes in Olympic or professional sports. A strong players' union combined with NFL management's lack of enthusiasm for a strong drug-testing program hindered the development of any comprehensive attack against drug use in the NFL. Some players have even charged that NFL team personnel often openly subvert the process, as an unnamed NFL player told *Sports Illustrated* (Wulf, 1991):

The problem is enforcement. Some clubs have a guy who enforces the testing. Our guy is like one of the boys. He sits by the weight room eating a sandwich. Say it's your turn to be tested. You say, "Pete, my urine's a little weak today, let me come back tomorrow," or you get the trainer to piss in the bottle for you and give Pete that one. It's a joke. (p. 10)

Olympic Hurdle—Volunteers

In the Olympic sports, the collection process presents a different hurdle to the effectiveness of drug testing. The collection of a urine sample from an athlete is an important first step in the drug-testing chain of custody. Almost universally, however, this process is operated by volunteers. Some may be well-trained medical professionals, others high school students. This reliance on volunteer help and the design of the collection process can create problems. In the celebrated case of Randy Barnes, testimony revealed what some consider a huge flaw in the collection process. According to documents and transcripts of Barnes's hearing before TAC (1990), the individual who served as the crew chief at the meet in Malmo, Sweden, where Barnes allegedly tested positive for methyltestosterone, (a) failed to list the envopack number for Barnes's sample on Barnes's form, and (b) possessed all the tools necessary to substitute another sample for the one Barnes had given and avoid detection of such a switch.

Alvin Chriss, former special assistant to the executive director of TAC, who was involved in drafting TAC's current drug-testing legislation, said:

One guy had control of everything. Whether or not I have a doubt that this man and his wife did in fact attempt to subvert the process, which I do not believe they did, the IAAF should not be allowed to defend the sloppiness of a procedure that allows this kind of work to pass muster. (Chriss, 1991)

As was noted in the Powell case described earlier in this chapter, mistakes in the process can invalidate a positive laboratory result and undermine the credibility of the system. Training for the volunteers who often play key roles in the collection process is often minimal and there is no formal review of the process.

The Media

From 1968 to 1988, sports drug testing developed from a cottage industry to an amorphous, semiregulated business largely out of the public view. Then Ben Johnson tested positive, and drug use and drug testing became front-page news in almost every media outlet in the world. The Dubin Inquiry grabbed the world's attention. Since Johnson was caught in Seoul, hardly a week goes by without some mention of drugs in sports. Until Johnson was caught, the media often ignored the issue, looked the other way, or merely believed drug stories were bad copy. The following excerpt from a column written by Alan Greenberg (1991) of the *Hartford Courant* is typical of many reporters' treatment of the issue:

I was covering the Los Angeles Raiders when Alzado, who had played previously with the Denver Broncos and Cleveland Browns, joined [the team] in 1982. He had acne on his back and upper arms, classic signs of steroid use. And his moods? One minute, he was the greatest guy in the world; the next minute, he was an erupting volcano for seemingly no reason.

In 1984, I was talking to one of his teammates across the Raiders' dressing room, when Alzado, with no provocation, picked up his gray metal stool and threw it in my direction, shouting something about "reporters in the locker room." Shaken, I asked several players who knew him best what was bugging him. They said Alzado had probably just had a steroid injection and to stay out of his way. Good advice.

A more sobering analysis was delivered by Greenberg's colleague Jerry Trecker (1991) of the *Hartford Courant*:

A sports machine capable of pretending that it doesn't debase the nation's educational system with its flaunting of academic standards, is equally adept at convincing itself that drug use really isn't that widespread. A sports media that pretends to birddog its subject by analyzing every play of a Super Bowl or an NCAA basketball final is also good at imagining that an occasional "expose" discharges the responsibility to truly profile the athletes it glorifies. And fans who may care more about the money they bet on a game than the way their favorites win are unlikely to insist upon high standards in the locker room.

Conclusion

The concept of analyzing an athlete's urine for the presence of prohibited substances seems simple. Just put the fluids into the machine and wait for the results. But, like everything else, what seems simple has a way of becoming complex. Machines fail. They are designed and operated by humans. Humans make mistakes. A mistake in a drug test can cost an athlete a medal or a career. Thus, much of the debate surrounding drug testing concerns ways to avoid those mistakes. Catch the cheaters, but don't ban an innocent man or woman.

This aversion to accusing the innocent is the rationale sports administrators cite when explaining the cloak of secrecy in drug testing. Test results are supposed to be private until a final determination is made on the guilt or innocence of the athlete. But there are leaks, rumors, and accusations of cover-ups that a system draped in confidentiality is ill equipped to deal with effectively.

Thus a process based on science becomes embroiled in human emotion. As TAC's executive director Ollan Cassell (1991) told a meeting of race directors, drug testing is one of the most emotional issues an athlete, coach, or sports administrator encounters because the stakes are so high.

It is complex because the research in the field is so new and limited to only a very select group of laboratories. Thus the seemingly simple question of whether or not an athlete is truly guilty of using a banned substance is often obscured by conflicting testimony, testimony that is often slanted for political or economic gain.

Although drug testing is offered as the solution to the problem of drug use by athletes, the system's effectiveness is directly related to the competence and integrity of those who operate it. Because of the high stakes involved, that competence and integrity will always be challenged. The key to evaluating the system's effectiveness, therefore, is how well its operators maintain their high standards in the face of the constant barrage of criticism directed at their operations.

In its infancy, drug testing was established as a deterrent to athletes using drugs. As the testing system enters adulthood, the burdens upon it have increased. Now, it is supposed to be a world-wide police agency, ferreting out cheaters and insuring a "level playing field." And it is to do this using the budget of a Third World country.

It is not hard to see why it is easier to find flaws in such an operation than it is to understand how far the system has grown in the past 30 years. With all its imperfections, it has accomplished a great deal. Like an adult, it is entering what could potentially be its most productive years. With all the publicity directed toward this system since the Seoul Olympics, the time appears to be right for the full maturation of the system. Drug testing is still a young science, and how it deals with its entry into adulthood may determine its ultimate role in the history of sport.

References

Almond, E. (1989, September 8). Colorado case fuels drug-testing furor. *Los Angeles Times*.

Almond, E. (1990, June 12). U.S. track group's drug enforcement in question. *Los Angeles Times*.

Armstrong, R. (1991, February 1). *The lessons learned from Canada's Dubin Inquiry*. Speech delivered at the International Symposium on Sport and Law, Monte Carlo.

Beckett, A.H., & Ljungqvist, A. (1989, June 5-7). Unpublished interview conducted at second International Athletic Foundation World Symposium on Doping in Sport, Monte Carlo.

Bedell, D. (1991, April 17). Athletes use a variety of methods to overcome drug tests. *Dallas Morning News*.

Biggane, B. (1991, August 22). Numerous ways around testing. Cox News Services.

Bilac back in business. (1991, July). *T & F News*, p. 50.

Black, D. (1991). Unpublished interview.

Boswell, R. (1988, June 27). World conference attacks illicit drugs. *The Ottawa Citizen*.

Bottomley, M. (1988). Report. In P. Bellotti, G. Benzi, & A. Ljungqvist (Eds.), *International Athletic Foundation World Symposium on Doping in*

Sport: Official Proceedings (pp. 209-211). Monte Carlo, Monaco: International Athletic Foundation.

Bouton, J. (1970). *Ball four*. Bell. (Revised in 1990 and published by Macmillan, New York)

Buffery, S., & Parrish, W. (1989, August 2). World body ignored positive drug tests & Doc rips "rescue." *Toronto Sun*.

Cassell, O. (1991, November 16). Speech delivered at Road Race Management Conference, Washington, DC.

Catlin, D.H. (1987). Detection of drug use by athletes. In R. Strauss (Ed.), *Drugs and performance in sports* (pp. 103-121). Philadelphia: Sanders.

Catlin, D.H. (1991). Unpublished interview.

Catlin, D.H., & Hatton, C.K. (1991). Use and abuse of anabolic and other drugs for athletic enhancement. *Advances in Internal Medicine, 36*, 399-424.

Catlin, D.H., Kammerer, R.C., Hatton, C.K., et al. (1987). Analytical chemistry at the Games of the XXIIIrd Olympiad in Los Angeles, 1984. *Clinical Chemistry, 33*, 319-327.

Catlin, D.H., & Moses, E. (1989). Unpublished interviews.

Chriss, A. (1990). Unpublished interview.

Chriss, A. (1991). Unpublished interview.

Court backs NCAA's drug tests. (1988, February 26). *St. Paul Pioneer Press*.

The death of Birgit Dressel. (1988, February/March). *Athletics*, pp. 6-10.

Demak, R., & Kirshenbaum, J. (1990, January). The NFL fails its drug test. *Sports Illustrated*.

de Merode, A. (1988, February). Unpublished telephone interview conducted during Winter Olympics.

Denton, H. (1989, March 5). Charlie Francis: The doctor is in. *Washington Post*.

DiPasquale, M. (1991). Polypharmacy: Anabolic steroids and beyond. *Drugs in Sports*, premier issue, pp. 2-3.

Donike, M., Geyer, H., Gotzmann, A., et al. (1988). Dope analysis. In P. Bellotti, G. Benzi, & A. Ljungqvist (Eds.), *International Athletic Foundation World Symposium on Doping in Sport: Official Proceedings* (pp. 53-80). Monte Carlo, Monaco: International Athletic Foundation.

Donohoe, T., & Johnson, N. (1986). *Foul play*. Oxford, England: Blackwell.

Doping tests. (1989, December 13). Associated Press wire service.

Down on dope. (1988, June 27). *Toronto Sun*, p. 80.

Drug tests sought. (1987, June 12). *Toronto Sun*.

Dubin, C.L. (1990). *Commission of inquiry into the use of drugs and banned practices intended to increase athletic performance*. Ottawa, ON: Canadian Government Publishing Centre.

Ferstle, J. (1991, August 18). U.S. authorities might have key player in drug network. *St. Paul Pioneer Press*.

Forbes, G. (1989, September 1). Steroids losers: Daringly foolish to try. *USA Today*.

Francis, C. (1991). Unpublished interview.

Gasbarrone, E., & Roasti, F. (1988). Report. In P. Bellotti, G. Benzi, & A. Ljungquist (Eds.), *International Athletic Foundation World Symposium on Doping in Sport: Official Proceedings* (pp. 222-224). Monte Carlo, Monaco: International Athletic Foundation.

Gasser v. Stinson (and another). (1988, June 15). Lexis Nexis case summary of decision.

Glauber, B. (1990, February 23). NFL's drug adviser resigns. *Newsday.*

Greenberg, A. (1991, June 29). Alzado has a serious message to kids about steroids—Don't use 'em. *Hartford Courant.*

Harvey, R. (1990, December 3). Magazine says East Germans used steroids. *Los Angeles Times.*

Hatton, C.K., & Catlin, D.H. (1987). Detection of androgenic anabolic steroids in urine. *Clinics in Laboratory Medicine, 7,* 655-668.

Hynes, M. (1988, June 28). Controls sought for drugs. *Globe and Mail.*

Hynes, M. (1988, June 29). Norway cracks down on steroids. *Globe and Mail.*

International Olympic Committee. (1973, June 18, July 12 & 13). *Investigative hearings on the proper and improper use of drugs by athletes.* Testimony before the U.S. Senate Judiciary Committee.

International Olympic Committee. (1989). Analytical results of A-samples at the games of the XXIVth Olympiad in Seoul, 1988. (IOC address: Chateau Vidy, CH-1007, Lausanne, Switzerland)

IOC-drugs. (1988, November 17). Associated Press wire service.

Janofsky, M., & Alfano, P. (1988, November 17). System accused of failing test posed by drugs. *New York Times,* p. 1, 45.

Kammerer, C. (1991). Unpublished interview.

Keisser, B. (1991, July 16). We need to pass Alzado's painful lesson on to the kids. Knight-Ridder News Service.

Kimmage, P. (1990). *A rough ride: An insight into pro cycling.* London: Stanley Paul.

Kirsch, A. (1988). Report. In P. Bellotti, G. Benzi, & A. Ljungquist (Eds.), *International Athletic Foundation World Symposium on Doping in Sport: Official Proceedings* (pp. 219-222). Monte Carlo, Monaco: International Athletic Foundation.

Labs under IOC gun. (1988, May 5). *Toronto Sun.*

Lambelet, D. (1989). Unpublished interviews.

Los Angeles Olympic Organizing Committee. (1985). *Official report of the games of the XXIIIrd Olympiad, Los Angeles, 1984* (2 vols.). Los Angeles: Author.

Mandell, A.J. (1976). *The nightmare season.* New York: Random House.

Marvez, A. (1991, July 21). WWF steroid plan likely to fail test. Knight-Ridder News Service.

Millen barred but U.S. plans to file appeal. (1989, April 22). *St. Paul Pioneer Press.*

Moses, E. (1989). Unpublished interview.

National Athletics Board of Review of The Athletics Congress. (1990, July 16). Decision of the NABR panel on the case of Charles R. DeBus (SP No. 1-07-07/1989).

Norman, N. (1988). Report. In P. Bellotti, G. Benzi, & A. Ljungquist (Eds.), *International Athletic Foundation World Symposium on Doping in Sport: Official Proceedings* (pp. 211-213). Monte Carlo, Monaco: International Athletic Foundation.

Park, J. (1989, June 5-7). *Review of the Seoul Laboratory activities—Seoul Olympic Games 1988.* Paper presented at the second International Athletic Foundation World Symposium on Doping in Sport, Monte Carlo, Monaco.

Patrick, D. (1989, June 20). Doctor's account confirms rumors. *USA Today.*

Plucknett v. TAC/USA. (1982, April 24). U.S. District Court for the Northern District of California, Palo Alto (Document No. C820545MHP).

Puffer, J. (1988, May). Unpublished interview conducted at American College of Sports Medicine annual meeting, Dallas.

Richmond-Tennant. (1990, February 20). Associated Press wire service.

Solberg wins damages. (1990, October 11). *Athletics Today,* p. 4.

Starcevic, N. (1990, December 3). Doping—East Germany. Associated Press wire service.

Stuart, H. (1988, June 27). Down on dope. *Toronto Sun*

The Athletics Congress. (1989). Decisions of hearing panels in cases of Augie Wolf and Billy Olsen.

The Athletics Congress. (1990, December 20). Official transcript of hearings: Application of Randy Barnes.

The Athletics Congress (TAC) Doping Control Review Board. (1991, October 4). Decision of DCRB in the case of Harry L. Reynolds. (TAC address: P.O. Box 120, Indianapolis, IN 46206)

Trecker, J. (1991, July 16). Sports continue without real concern for drug abuse. *Hartford Courant.*

United States Olympic Committee. (1987). Unpublished letters from George Miller and Ollan Cassell. (USOC address: 1750 E. Boulder St., Colorado Springs, CO 80909)

Update: Drug testing out. (1989, August 23). *USA Today.*

Videman, T. (1989, June 5-7). Speech delivered at second International Athletic Foundation World Symposium on Doping in Sport, Monte Carlo, Monaco.

Von vorn bis hinten belogen. (1992, February 10). *Der Spiegel.*

Voy, R. (1988). Unpublished interview.

Voy, R., & Deeter, K.D. (1991). *Drugs, sport, and politics: The inside story about drug use in sport and its political cover-up, with a prescription for reform.* Champaign, IL: Leisure Press.

Wadler, G.I., & Hainline, B. (1989). *Drugs and the athlete.* Philadelphia: Davis.

Warshaw, A. (1989, October 12). Doping. Associated Press Wire Service.

Wilson, S. (1991, April 16). IOC meetings. Associated Press sportswire.

Wimbledon-drugs. (1990, June 24). Associated Press wire service.

Wong, G. (1988). *Essentials of amateur sports law*. Dover: Auburn House.

Wulf, S. (Ed.) (1991, July 22). Scorecard: Eye openers. *Sports Illustrated*, p. 10.

Yesalis, C.E. (1991). Personal communication.

Zanca, S. (1991, February 12). Figure skating—Drugs. Associated Press Wire Service.